Hammond's Choice

Most of the things we decide are not what we know to be best. We say yes, merely because we are driven into a corner and must say something.

—Frank Crane

PROLOGUE

She had always considered herself a patient person. Rome wasn't built in a day: one step at a time. Good things take a long time. These clichés made sense to her and she felt pride in her ability to set personal goals and methodically achieve them. Obstacles in her course did not bother her. She would patiently figure out how to get around or remove whatever stood in her way. When the obstruction was a person she would smile and calmly persist until the individual realized she was not going away and would step aside.

But this was different. She had waited so long she sometimes wondered if it would ever happen. But when it did happen, when her beautiful baby was ready to be delivered, she knew it had been worth every minute of anxious anticipation.

Drawing upon a reserve beyond the wall of fatigue that had fallen on her, she bore down and pushed with all of her might. Her face turned crimson, the cords in her neck looked as if they would snap, but she kept pushing. Even when the doctor told her he was out, even after her baby uttered his first cry, she was reluctant to stop pushing, afraid her son might become stuck. It took the gentle touch of a nurse to convince her to let go. Placing a warm hand on her brow, the nurse whispered into her ear, it's okay, he's arrived, he's with you now.

She looked up and saw her husband dressed in a green paper gown and cap, holding a tiny red-faced infant swaddled in a pale blue blanket. Even through her exhaustion she could see her son's distinctive features: a surprising patch of thick black hair, wrinkled ears pressed against the side of his head, and dark eyes that seemed to be searching for her.

Backlit by the bright lights of the operating room, her husband and son appeared to be surrounded by a halo. She took a deep breath and exhaled, allowing herself to enjoy the sight of the two most important men in her life. At that moment she felt her heart might burst. She had just experienced a miracle and the love she felt for her husband and son were so intense the only thing she could do was to cry.

That image, so vivid and sustaining, would remain with her a long time, resurfacing at special as well as ordinary moments: Giving her infant son a bath and listening to his squeals of delight as she bathed his smooth, pink body, she would remember the three of them in the delivery room. Stifling a giggle as she watched her husband struggling to assemble the portable swing the instructions had promised could be put together in less than five minutes, she remembered how calm he seemed to be in the delivery room. For years, the image of her husband holding their newborn son filled her with love and hope and the sense that their life was whole.

Looking back, she sometimes wondered which had begun to fall apart first: the image or the reality. She eventually concluded that it didn't matter, though she desperately tried to hold on to both, even after the halo had faded and she began to question whether it was, in fact, a miracle that God had bestowed upon her the day Tommy was born.

CHAPTER ONE

On my last day at Kuperstein Discreet Surveillance, my supervisor, Mr. Gresh, a man of few words, called me into his office and shared his appraisal of my performance: "Neatness and cleanliness: B; ability to judge character: C-; perseverance: B+; physical and mental toughness: D-; technical skills: C-; able to follow directions: D; overall competence: C-. I hope you'll be a better graduate student than you were an investigator."

I was confident that I would. Not only could I make better use of my intellectual ability, but the prospect of conducting research in social psychology was a lot more appealing than sitting in a car waiting for our client's husband to show up at his mistress' mobile home. Besides, Syracuse University was more than four hundred miles from Toledo and the watchful eye of my mother. It had taken me awhile, but at thirty-seven I was finally on the right path.

Nearly two years later, as I struggled to finish my master's thesis, I wasn't so confident.

I had spent the morning in the computer lab mulling over my thesis data. Although I hadn't made much progress on the statistical analysis, sitting at the computer gazing into cyberspace for three hours had definitely stimulated my appetite. I decided to go to Cosmo's. Their pizza was good and the price was right. I was finishing my second slice when I saw a heavy man in a cream-colored poplin windbreaker push open the front door and walk into the pizzeria.

Definitely not my day, I thought as I watched the last person I wanted to see wade into the small crowd of students standing in the aisle.

Professor Mike Singleton was a study in contrasts. On the inside he

1

was neat, organized and extremely sharp. He had a photographic memory and an analytic mind that could, with equal ease, perform a complex non-parametric statistical computation or formulate the relationship between the savings and loan industry collapse and the absence of age-appropriate role expectations for children of the Kennedy era.

On the outside he was anything but neat. At five foot eight inches and more than two hundred pounds, he could best be described as rotund. His frizzy red hair was rarely cut and never combed, and his manner of dress was unique. He seemed to take pride in creating unusual combinations of color and patterns: A yellow and red striped shirt with black and white checked slacks one day might be followed by an orange shirt with brown polka dots, whose shirttail fell almost to the knees of his electric blue rayon trousers. If the occasion called for it, he might add a bright crimson tie from his alma mater, Harvard.

Singleton's wife, Mary, who is a master of understatement, once characterized his mode of dress as primitive eclecticism.

The professor's unorthodox appearance did little to detract from his popularity with students. He was one of the most highly rated teachers on campus and his course on the *Social Psychology of Late 20th Century Courting Behavior and Other Peculiar Human Rituals* was always oversubscribed. Graduate students pleaded with him to serve as their advisor. One student was so anxious to have Singleton as his mentor he offered to work as a research assistant without pay for a full year.

Like all great teachers, Singleton's strength lay not only in the amount of knowledge he possessed but in the passion with which he approached the subject matter. Standing in front of the lecture hall, trying to explain the concept of cognitive dissonance to a group of undergraduate students, Professor Singleton would become so excited that his hands would begin to quiver and his bushy red hair would bounce up and down.

As much as I liked and admired Professor Singleton, I definitely did not want to see him today. More accurately, I did not want him to see me.

A week ago I had assured him . . . no, *promised* him I would complete the analysis of my thesis data and have a first draft of the results written by today. My intentions were good, but my follow-through was weak. Last night, after a week of intense procrastination, I had been fully prepared to drive over to the computer lab and crunch some numbers. Then I was going to prepare a concise report of the results of my study, which undoubtedly would be acclaimed as a major scientific breakthrough in the field of social psychology.

Unfortunately, just as I was about to leave my apartment, my girlfriend Ollie had called to invite me over to her place for a brief visit. We were having some problems and I really needed to concentrate on my thesis. I told her I would catch up with her later. After I hung up I told myself I wasn't reverting to my typical mode of procrastination, that I really had to focus on my data. I almost convinced myself.

I had deliberately chosen Cosmo's because I knew Singleton was a man of habit. And he detested pizza. Every day at noon he walked down to the Varsity Restaurant, ordered a chicken salad sandwich on rye and a diet Coke, which he proceeded to devour in less than three minutes. He then returned to his office where he would read the latest issue of one of the many psychology journals to which he subscribed before walking up the hill to teach his one o'clock class.

I had clearly overestimated the strength of Singleton's habit.

That was my second mistake.

Watching the professor squeeze through the cluster of students, I slouched down in the booth, hoping he wouldn't see me. With any luck, his overstuffed briefcase would be jostled from his arms, spilling papers and books onto the floor. While Singleton frantically tried to retrieve his belongings I would quietly slip out of the booth and escape.

Apparently I was not going to have any luck today. Clutching his briefcase to his chest, Singleton wove through the crowd at what was for him warp speed.

"Ah, Martin," Singleton said, pulling up next to my booth. "I was hoping to find you here."

Realizing there was no way to escape, I opted for the next best alternative. "I know you're disappointed in me. I have no excuse to offer. I planned to do it and I didn't. That's all there is to it."

Knowing that Singleton was fond of Rotter's theory of locus of control, I hoped that my admission of culpability, my willingness to accept responsibility for my own actions (or lack of action in this instance) would temper his disappointment.

To my surprise, Professor Singleton did not appear to be interested in either my thesis or my locus of control.

"Do you have a moment?" Singleton asked. Dropping his briefcase on the table, he slid into the seat across from me. He didn't wait for a reply to his question. "I just came from a discussion with Dr. Barker, a colleague of mine. You may know Dr. Barker. He teaches in the clinical psychology division. He told me of a very troubling situation with one of his clients. I thought you might be able to help him."

I had heard of Dr. Barker but had not met him. Usually I tried to avoid the clinical psychology program. The clinical graduate students had a reputation of being more intense, more competitive than those in other divisions. If I were a clinician—which I am not and have no desire to be—I might have described their behavior as neurotic. From my limited experience with the faculty in the clinical program they served as pretty good role models for their protégés.

Professor Barker, on the other hand, had a solid reputation. By all accounts he was a dedicated teacher, skilled therapist, and competent researcher. Even more important, he appeared to be a fair and reasonable man who never missed an SU basketball home game.

For all those reasons, plus the fact that responding to Professor Singleton's request for help would postpone the inevitable embarrassing confrontation about my thesis work, I decided to pursue his request.

"What kind of trouble?" I asked.

"It's quite complicated," Singleton responded. "I think it would be better if you spoke directly to Dr. Barker."

"Okay," I said, trying to suppress my glee about the prospect of escaping unscathed. "What would be the best way of reaching Dr. Barker?"

"I knew I could count on you, Martin. Based on the probability that I would find you and you would be gracious enough to be willing to assist him, I arranged for Dr. Barker to be in his office at one forty-five, right after his psychotherapy seminar. He's in room 327 of the old Good Shepherd Hospital on University Avenue. He'll be expecting you."

Professor Singleton slid out of the booth and glanced at his watch. "That gives you twenty minutes, Martin. Please be prompt." Then he picked up his briefcase and walked quickly toward the exit, pushing his way through the crowd of waiting students.

Watching him waddle down the aisle, I realized, once again, what a masterful psychologist he was. Without saying a word he had managed to stoke my guilt to bonfire proportions, while at the same time presenting me with a clear path from the flames to a cool, inviting channel of redemption—helping Dr. Barker with his dilemma. Shaking my head in awe, I picked up a slice of pepperoni pizza from the plate and took a large bite.

The pizza was cold.

The old Good Shepherd Hospital was actually not very old. Built after World War II, its glass and chrome facade gave it a contemporary appearance. It had once served as a rehabilitation hospital, but the movement toward outpatient care and the erection of the huge Upstate Medical Center several blocks away had rendered the hospital obsolete.

With the student infirmary located on the first floor, the building retained its status as a health care facility. The second and third stories were occupied by the clinical psychology and counseling graduate programs. There was a standing joke that the infirmary had been strategically placed to serve as a safety net for students who came within harm's way of the graduate degree programs.

No one had ever refuted this theory.

When the weather was bad, which was most of the time in Syracuse, one could enter through Huntington Hall, directly across the street from Cosmos. Huntington Hall (also a former hospital) was built perpendicular to Good Shepherd. At the far left end of Huntington Hall was an indoor walkway that allowed one to enter the Good Shepherd Building without battling the elements.

Today was one of those days I decided to take advantage of the sheltered route. It was a blustery April day with the temperature in the forties and a steady drizzle that seemed to blow directly into my face regardless of which way I was facing.

Although I grew up in the Northeast—Teaneck, New Jersey to be precise—I was not prepared for the long, hard winters of central New York. The snow often started in October and usually didn't stop until the end of April. One spring I celebrated Memorial Day with an abbreviated snowball fight at a picnic on the northern shore of Onondaga Lake. We had just finished a huge meal of Italian sausage, Polish sausage and American hamburger (even then we were culturally diverse) and were walking in the woods when we discovered a large mound of unmelted snow.

I don't think I'll ever become accustomed to Syracuse weather.

Dr. Matthew Barker was waiting for me at the entrance to his office. He was a small, thin man with narrow shoulders who obviously paid a lot of attention to his appearance. His black hair had a few gray streaks at the temples and was neatly layered to make his narrow head seem wider. He wore a navy blue cashmere blazer over a blue pinstripe shirt and an imported burgundy silk tie with a muted floral design. His charcoal flannel slacks had a crisp crease and his black leather Italian loafers were freshly polished.

The only thing about him that wasn't totally neat and smooth was his forehead, which had several deep wrinkles. In spite of his furrowed brow his face had an aura of tranquility. As he shook my hand my immediate reaction was to let down my guard and tell him about the awful day I was having.

At that moment, looking into his pale blue eyes, I understood why he had such an excellent reputation as a therapist.

"It was kind of you to meet with me at such short notice," Barker said in a voice as mellow as Manilow. "Please make yourself comfortable," he said, gesturing toward a dark blue Lazy Boy recliner.

Looking at the plush chair with its thick cushion, I felt a twinge of anxiety. Was I actually afraid that if I sank into one of those chairs I would blurt out my deep, dark secrets? My reaction was particularly frightening since, as far as I knew, I didn't have any secrets that were deeper and darker than my failure to write up my thesis results.

I controlled my anxiety and sat in the chair farthest from Dr. Barker. He pulled a small gray tweed armchair away from the wall and placed it at a right angle to mine. Easing himself slowly into the chair he pressed together the palms of his hands and rested his chin on his fingertips. "Did Mike tell you anything about my client's problem?" he asked.

"No, Professor Singleton said it would be better if you explained it to me." It was difficult switching roles. As a student I always called Singleton

6

"Professor" or "Doctor". All of his students did in spite of his casual, informal manner. I guess we were awestruck by his incredible mind and the wealth of knowledge he possessed. Now, in my role as investigator, in the presence of another faculty member, I was unsure of how to refer to him.

I chose the safer alternative.

Barker gazed at me for a moment. I wondered whether he was reading my mind. He seemed so perceptive. Maybe he was having second thoughts about asking a graduate student, an *ambivalent* graduate student no less, to help his client. I waited anxiously, expecting the worst.

Finally, Barker lowered his hands to his lap. "You understand, of course, that the rules of confidentiality apply here," he said softly.

I nodded.

"This is a delicate matter. My clients have asked me to assist them. But until they sign a release indicating their willingness to give information to you, I am limited in my ability to share with you specific details of their situation."

I knew about confidentiality from the correspondence course on private investigation I took several years ago while doing an apprenticeship with a well-known investigatory agency. I quit the job shortly after I completed the apprenticeship—there were too many rules and restrictions— but I passed the course and qualified for my license.

I also knew about therapist-client confidentiality from a course on abnormal psychology I had taken, but I didn't understand how that actually worked.

"What I will do," Barker said, "is describe the situation in hypothetical terms, leaving out any identifying information. If you decide that you might be able to help and my clients express interest in retaining you, I will have them sign a release so I may put you in touch with them."

It sounded complicated, but what did I know. I was a mere social psychology graduate student, not at all well-versed in the practice of psychotherapy. "You mentioned *clients,*" I said. "From my discussion with Professor Singleton I was under the impression there was only one client." I hoped that Barker noticed my perceptiveness.

"Let's say that we're speaking about a couple, a husband and wife." Barker was obviously not impressed. "Let's say this couple has a son.

They're both in their mid-thirties when the boy is born and he quickly becomes the center of their universe. As an infant he is cute and bubbly and almost always happy. A simple smile from him melts his parents' hearts. But as this boy grows older he changes. He does not enjoy the company of others, becomes quite upset when his routine is disturbed, and sometimes strikes out unpredictably, smashing his toys or anything else within his reach."

I wondered where he was going with all of this. I hoped he didn't expect me to work with this child. Surely Professor Singleton had told them I wasn't on the helping side of psychology.

"The parents are frantic," he continued. "They don't understand why this has happened. They turn to professionals for help, but no one is even able to give them a good explanation of why their sweet little boy is so unhappy and explosive. The boy's behavior continues to deteriorate. At first they hold out hope that this is a passing phase, a normal stage of development. Eventually they can no longer avoid the truth: their son has serious emotional problems, so serious in fact that he requires intensive treatment in a setting where he can be supervised twenty-four hours a day."

"You mean like a psychiatric hospital?"

"No. He has been stabilized, at least to the extent that he can be," Barker explained. "This child, or I should say adolescent, since he's fourteen years old, would be in a residential treatment center which provides a comprehensive therapeutic milieu."

"Therapeutic milieu?" I asked, once again showing my ignorance.

"I'm sorry," Barker said, smiling apologetically. "I assumed that since you were in psychology you would be familiar with our jargon. Sometimes I think we create terminology just to make sure that people outside our profession can't understand our field and need us to translate the jargon for them; sort of a job security ploy on our part. Anyway, therapeutic milieu is a fancy term for using the setting where a person eats, works and plays as a means for helping him or her deal with their problems. By structuring all of the elements of the living situation—people, activities, even the physical space—into a positive, supportive learning environment, mental health professionals believe they can help persons with mental disorders function better. Clinicians use the milieu to help residents increase their social and daily living skills, learn more effective ways to cope with stress and enhance their self-esteem."

"Oh, I get it. Like the program they used in *A Clockwork Orange*."

Barker smiled. "Touché, Mr. Fenton. I suppose I deserve that for being so esoteric. Actually milieu programs can be quite effective if those in charge avoid the typical institutional pitfalls."

"Translate, please," I liked that Barker was able to acknowledge his own shortcomings. I was beginning to feel more at ease with him.

"Sorry again," he chuckled. "What I meant to say is that all therapeutic interventions, including milieu programs, should always be focused on one overriding purpose: to return the person to their natural environment, to their community and, if at all possible, to their own home. Unfortunately it is too easy for staff in a restrictive setting, like a hospital or residential treatment center, to forget that goal. Since institutions almost always act to perpetuate themselves, there is a risk that the staff will be more concerned about protecting the established order than helping the client function in the community."

"Is that what's happened to this hypothetical adolescent?"

"I don't really know much about the program he's in, but that's not the reason his parents need help. This particular boy has a very serious problem."

"But what can I do to help?" I asked, feeling confused, "I'm not trained in clinical psychology."

"I know, Mr. Fenton. This youngster's problems are beyond the realm of psychology."

"What do you mean?"

Barker cleared his throat and leaned forward. "The boy we're speaking about has been accused of killing one of the other children in the program."

CHAPTER TWO

*Too many staff. And who are these other people? They should
go away. Just leave me alone. I'm tired. I don't feel good.
Leave me alone.*

I felt as if I were standing in a warm shower and the water suddenly
turned ice-cold. "Jesus," I said, sucking in my breath. "Did you say
killed?"

"I'm afraid so," Barker replied. His pale blue eyes now looked sad.
"You can imagine how shocked his parents were when they were told. I
worked with the boy several years ago and even though I knew he had
some serious problems I was stunned by the news." He paused and looked
up at the ceiling. With his brow furrowed even more than it had been, he
appeared to be deep in thought. After a few seconds he lowered his head
and looked directly into my eyes. "I'm tempted to tell you more, but I
don't want to compromise the family's confidentiality. Do you think you
would be willing to talk to them, to see if you might be able to help?"

"I . . . I don't know. This is a little bit out of my league. I've dealt with
adultery, insurance scams . . . even a missing person, once. But *murder*.
That's a whole different category. Don't they have a lawyer?"

Barker shook his head slowly. "It's a complicated situation, Marty,"
he said. "I know you're not a seasoned veteran. But Mike speaks highly
of you. He says you're bright and perceptive, that you have an uncanny
knack for solving puzzles. He also says you have a strong sense of justice,
especially when it comes to the underdog. Mike's recommendation means
a lot to me."

His flattery rendered me speechless. It was true that I have a knack
for puzzles, always have. When I was a kid I would work on anything

I could get my hands on: crosswords, jigsaws, and anagrams. It didn't matter what type of puzzle it was as long as it distracted me from my mother's constant prodding.

After awhile I did puzzles even when my mother wasn't nudging me. Now, even though I live several hundred miles away from my mother, I continue to be a puzzle junkie.

Aside from his comment about being good at puzzles, I didn't recognize anything in Barker's statement that resembled me. I consider myself to be an ordinary person. True, I am a little older than your average graduate student, but that's not an achievement likely to get me inducted into the Sherlock Holmes Hall of Fame.

Either Professor Singleton saw something in me that I wasn't aware of, or he was once again playing with my mind, trying to persuade me to help Dr. Barker.

I was betting on his prowess as a psychologist.

But it really didn't matter.

"Okay," I said reluctantly. "I'll give it a shot."

"Very good," Barker responded, giving me a warm smile. He seemed relieved. "I don't anticipate any complications with my clients. I'll speak with them later this afternoon and get back to you this evening if that's okay with you."

"Sure, I should be home after nine." This was the night I worked as a volunteer tutor at Huntington Family Center. I was usually finished by eight-thirty and home by nine.

"I'll call you by ten," Barker said. "Mike told me you're working hard to complete your thesis. I wouldn't want to keep you from your scholarly pursuit."

He spoke in a matter-of-fact manner. There was no hint of irony in his voice, no indication that he was poking fun at me.

But the small curl in his lip told me clearly that the good Professor Singleton had briefed Dr. Barker on my procrastinating ways.

Professor Barker's reference to my academic work habits didn't have a significant effect on my productivity. After I left his office I went directly to the library, hoping to complete the first draft of the results section of my thesis. Several hours of staring at computer printouts of statistical data failed to inspire me but left me with an awful headache. In a desperate act of self-deception, I scribbled a few notes, threw my mostly blank notepad into my canvas briefcase and walked down to the Varsity Restaurant, where I consoled myself with a large taco salad and a frozen yogurt shake; comfort food for the twenty-first century. Driving home, I resolved to get up early the next morning and work until I completed the results chapter. After all, I had done all the hard parts: developed the proposal, conducted the interviews, and analyzed the data. All that remained was to put the damn thing down on paper, which was no big deal.

By the time I reached my apartment building I felt better. My frustration had subsided and my confidence was restored.

Self-deception used sparingly is a marvelous psychic tonic.

I heard my telephone ringing as I reached the top of the landing. I hurried down the corridor, fumbled for my key ring, found the key to the apartment, and quickly unlocked the door. I pushed open the door and rushed to the kitchen.

As I reached for the handset, the ringing stopped.

I stood next to the kitchen counter, listening to the dial tone, and tried to guess who had called. It might have been my mother, calling to tell me that I needed to make contact with my sister, but actually intending to remind me that I hadn't written or called her (my mother) often enough. Or it could have been Ollie, anxious to tell me she couldn't stand being without me for another moment. Probably not her, I thought, conjuring up a pleasing mental image of the two of us locked in a passionate embrace.

Maybe it was Professor Singleton, checking in to see if his subtle, guilt-inducing strategy had motivated me to do some work on my thesis.

Glancing at my Casio I saw that it was a few minutes after nine P.M. Most likely the person on the other end of the line had been Dr. Barker, calling to let me know the outcome of his conversation with his clients, the parents of the accused boy.

There was an easy way to find out who had called, but I was reluctant to use it.

After several moments of futile guessing I conceded that my clairvoyant powers were not up to the task of identifying the caller I had missed. I punched in the seven familiar numbers and held the telephone receiver away from my ear.

Not far enough. The hacking cough grated on my ear, making me wince. "Good evening, this is Mr. Fenton's service," Mrs. D managed to blurt out before breaking into another coughing jag.

Mrs. D was one of the premier operators for the We-Care Answering Service. Several times I had been on the verge of terminating my relationship with We-Care, but my intense dislike of answering machines and the need to be accessible to the few people who actually wanted to contact me had kept me from dropping their service.

"Good evening, Mrs. D," I said politely, hoping I would not trigger another coughing spell. "How are you feeling, today?"

"Oh, Mr. Fenton, you're such a nice man, always concerned about the welfare of your operators. I wish some of our other clients were half as considerate as you. I suppose you would like to know who left messages for you, today."

"That would be nice, Mrs. D."

"Let me see. I had your stack here a moment ago. Someone called for you just before you checked in."

I could hear her cough in the background as she searched for my messages. I had never been to the We-Care office—I was afraid that I might become too attached if I actually saw the operators—but I imagined a dingy room with peeling plaster and a single naked light bulb hanging from the ceiling. In my fantasy the operator on duty sat in an old swivel chair with a small, round back, facing a large old fashioned telephone console complete with head sets and patch cords. Mrs. D and the other operators sat waist deep in a pile of pink telephone message slips. The old messages were never thrown out. They were simply covered over by the next day's batch.

It was a wonder they ever found a message.

"Okay, I think I have all of them," she said, struggling to catch her breath. "Oh my goodness, how disappointing. That nice woman, Mrs. Fenton, your mother, didn't call today."

One thing I could say in their favor was that the We-Care operators definitely took a personal interest in their work. Once Mrs. O, whose telephone voice bore a faint resemblance to Marilyn Monroe with a cheek full of chewing tobacco, began to weep when she told me that Ollie had

13

called to say she had to work late and could not meet me for dinner.

"What are my messages, Mrs. D?"

"Oh, you only have one message, Mrs. Fenton. A Mr . . . . excuse me, Dr. Barker called. He left a number and said you can call him any time before midnight."

I thanked Mrs. D and was about to hang up when she gasped my name between two coughs that may have registered on the Richter scale.

"Ms. Tolliver also called . . ."

"I thought you said there was only one message," I said, feeling slightly annoyed at her carelessness.

"There was," she replied. "Ms. Tolliver said there was no message, that she would call you later."

Dr. Barker answered on the second ring. He told me he had talked with the parents of the boy accused of killing another resident of the treatment center. He must have done a good job of promoting me. The parents, Ruth and Larry Hammond, wanted to meet with me as soon as possible. They asked Dr. Barker to have me call them that night. I thanked the professor and told him I would keep in touch.

Larry Hammond answered the telephone. He had a deep, resonant voice, one of those Midwestern announcer voices that I associated with movie newsreels and documentary films. It wasn't until later, when I got to know Larry Hammond, that I was able to detect the trace of sadness in his voice. One had to listen closely to hear it, but it was always there.

After listening to how grateful Hammond was that I had agreed to help them, I asked when we could discuss his son's problem. We agreed to meet the next day for breakfast at the Hammonds' home in Liverpool.

I dialed Ollie's number, hoping she was not at the University's sculpture studio where she spent a couple of evenings a week. Although she had a master's degree in fine arts, the closest she had come to finding a position in her field was at the gift shop of the Everson Museum. Manager of the gift shop was not exactly what Ollie had in mind when she set out from the academy, sheepskin in one hand, sculpture tools in the other, ready to dazzle the world of art with her knowledge and talent. The only thing that kept her at the Everson—besides the meager salary that allowed her to pay the rent on her apartment—was the faint hope that Dr. Halverman or Mrs. Wonderby, the museum's assistant curators, might finally retire, giving her a shot at a legitimate art job. Everyone I spoke to who knew anything about art told me Ollie was brilliant, that she had learned more about the fine arts in her dozen years of involvement than the two incumbents had acquired in their combined experience of more than seventy-five years.

Unfortunately the two elderly assistant curators gave no indication of retiring and Ollie was too nice to imagine an alternative way they might vacate their positions. So Ollie toiled patiently in the gift shop during the day and spent her evenings creating graceful forms from large blocks of wood and stone.

That is, when she wasn't working out in preparation for an out-of-town bodybuilding competition. In addition to her other noteworthy attributes, Ollie had an incredible body. Not one of those over-developed, muscle-bound physiques you sometimes see on television, but a taut, athletic body with just enough muscle definition to dissuade anyone who might consider kicking sand in her direction.

Ollie defied the stereotype of a female bodybuilder in other ways also. She was quite modest. Not only did she go to great lengths to conceal her well-endowed physique, she also refused to compete in any competition within a hundred miles of Syracuse. When she did compete, it took considerable coaxing and cajoling to find out how she placed, even though she often did well.

After a half dozen rings, I concluded that she wasn't home. As I hung up the receiver, I congratulated myself for reacting so calmly. A year ago I would have been upset that Ollie wasn't waiting with great anticipation for me. My imagination would have conjured up a host of vivid scenarios; in each, Ollie would be intensely engaged with a tall handsome man. And they weren't discussing sculpture.

Now, however, I was able to accept the fact that Ollie was not at home without punishing myself with fantasies of her with other men. Our relationship had come a long way since last year and I felt good about that. I'm not suggesting that things were perfect, but they were much better.

So much better that I only had to complete one crossword puzzle before I was able to suppress the impulse to jump into my car and drive to the sculpture studio.

Liverpool is noted for several things: Heid's Hot Dogs, the huge General Electric plant that has employed thousands of central New Yorkers for many generations and the fact that it bears the same name as the seaport city in western England that was the home of the Beatles. It also has the reputation of being a fairly convenient, though dull, suburb located less than a ten minute drive from the heart of downtown Syracuse.

The Hammonds lived in a nineteen-fifties brick ranch on a quiet cul-de-sac of almost identical houses. I parked my Honda on the street and thanked it for completing another trip, short as it was, without breaking down. Walking on the flagstone path leading to their front door, I tried to imagine how such a wholesome looking environment could spawn a young boy capable of murdering another child.

Larry Hammond greeted me with a tight-lipped smile that looked as if it had taken a lot of energy to produce. He was a heavyset man with a full head of thick black hair and bushy eyebrows that came together above his nose. He wore a dark brown suit, a white broadcloth shirt, and a nineties tie with a bright floral pattern.

"Thank you for coming out on such short notice," he said, shaking my hand firmly. "Can I get you a cup of coffee or some juice?"

I declined his offer and he led me into a small living room filled with early American furniture. Ruth Hammond, a petite black-haired woman who appeared to be in her early forties, sat in the middle of a brown tweed high-backed sofa. She was dressed in a long-sleeved navy blue dress with a maroon silk scarf draped over her shoulders. In her lap she held a large green photo album. The album was open and she appeared to be running her fingers in a circular motion over one of the photographs.

I held out my hand as I approached her. Without rising, she took it and said she was pleased to meet me. I tried to make eye contact with her but she kept her eyes down, looking at the photo album.

"Is that your son?" I asked.

She looked up and seemed startled to see me. "Yes, that's Tommy when he was much younger." She handed the album to me. There were four pictures on the page, each featuring a small dark-haired boy. In one picture he sat in a high chair, his face covered with icing from a piece of cake, the remains of which appear to have been used to decorate the tray of his chair. There was a picture of him sitting in his mother's lap playing patty cake. And another showed his father bent over helping him to navigate his tricycle. In the last picture he was by himself dressed in a little sailor suit. I'm not good at estimating children's ages, but I would guess that those photos were taken when he was between the ages of one and three. In all of the photos he had the same crooked smile and it was obvious from their expressions that his parents adored him.

"Cute little boy," I remarked. No response.

"I understand you need someone to do some investigating," I said, trying to ease the tension—my tension, at least.

"To say that we need someone to investigate might be an understatement," Larry Hammond said, with his forced smile. "We're actually pretty desperate at this point." He gestured for me to sit in a wing chair opposite the sofa. He sat next to his wife. For a big man, Hammond moved gracefully. I guessed that he had been an athlete in his youth. "Dr. Barker tells me he explained our problem to you," Mr. Hammond said.

"That's right," I said. "I'm sorry to have to meet you under such disturbing circumstances, but I'm going to do my best to help you. When was the last time you spoke to your son?"

The Hammonds looked at each other. This time it was Mrs. Hammond who spoke. "I guess Dr. Barker didn't tell you everything." She wrung her hands as she spoke. "Tommy is a very disturbed boy. He's had serious emotional problems since he was a small child. In the beginning we thought he was just overactive, but—"

"Ruth is being kind," Larry interjected. "She knew that his outbursts were not normal long before I was willing to admit it."

"Let's not replay history," Ruth said. There was an edge to her voice that surprised me considering her husband had just acknowledged that she knew something was wrong with Tommy long before he was willing to accept that his son had a problem.

Larry closed his eyes for an instant, then proceeded to tell me about Tommy's behavior as a young child. In a detached, almost clinical manner, he described Tommy's sudden transformation from a docile little boy playing with his toys to a wild animal, flailing and screaming, froth forming at the corners of his mouth as he tore up books and threw model cars against the wall.

Or even worse.

"I had just returned from a business trip," Larry said. "It had been a tough trip, but a good one. This was when I still made an honest living as an electrical engineer at GE. Before they kicked me upstairs to a management position. We were bidding on a big military contract—I think it was the Navy—and I had been sent to St. Louis to work with some of our people there on the technical details of the proposal. It was a real killer. We had three days to put the whole thing together and we worked our tails off to meet the deadline. Even pulled an all-nighter, like we used to at college—"

"Mr. Fenton isn't interested in your autobiography, Larry," Ruth said, shaking her head slowly.

Larry glanced at her and for an instant seemed as if he was going to say something, but then turned back to me and continued his story.

"Tommy was seven at the time. He didn't like it when I went away, but on this particular occasion he hadn't given Ruth a hard time and seemed happy to see me. I gave him the little present I had picked up for him at the airport and played with him for a few minutes. Then we sat down to eat dinner."

Ruth shifted in her seat, turning away from Larry and toward the window. I couldn't tell if this was an attempt to shut out a painful memory or another expression of her irritation with Larry. The undercurrent of tension between the two of them was making me uncomfortable.

"We were all pretty hungry," Larry continued. "We ate quickly and did not talk. After a few minutes I asked Tommy to tell me about his school project. Tommy did not respond, but kept on eating. Ruth, who was sitting next to Tommy, tapped him on the shoulder and asked him again to tell me what he was doing.

"Suddenly Tommy leaped out of his chair and lunged at Ruth. He put his hands around her throat and started to choke her. It happened so quickly that neither of us was prepared. Ruth started to scream and I sat frozen in my seat, too stunned to react. It seemed unreal, as if I were watching a three-dimensional film projected onto our dining room table.

"Finally I came to my senses and tried to pull Tommy off Ruth. She had fallen from her chair and they were both on the ground. I reached down, put my hand on Tommy's shoulder and shook him, but he didn't let go. Then I grabbed him by the upper arm and tugged. He still didn't budge. By this time Ruth was turning red. Her calls for help came out as hissing whispers. I reached under Tommy's arms and pulled as hard as I could, but still could not get him to release his grip. I couldn't believe how strong he was. He couldn't have weighed more than fifty pounds but he seemed to have the strength of a two-hundred pound man.

"I started to feel my own strength fade and began to panic. What if I couldn't get Tommy off? Would he actually strangle Ruth? How could this be happening? I felt nauseated but knew I couldn't waste even a few seconds. Finally I grabbed Tommy by his tiny wrists, and with all my remaining strength, managed to pry his fingers loose. I yanked him backward and we landed on the floor, Tommy on his back, on top of me, swinging his arms and kicking his legs wildly while I lay there gasping for air, my arms wrapped around his waist holding on for dear life."

Larry was breathing heavily, as if he were reliving the awful scene he was describing. Ruth started at the wall, moving her head back and forth slowly. There were tears in her eyes.

Larry took a deep breath and exhaled. "I'll never forget that night. I'd never seen Tommy act like that and I was totally unprepared. For a moment I thought he was really going to kill Ruth and I wasn't going to be able to stop him. The whole thing didn't make sense to me. This was my son, my seven-year-old, fifty-pound little boy. What was he doing kneeling on my wife's chest, screaming like a primitive beast as he tried to strangle her? Why couldn't I—a two-hundred pound man—stop him?"

I was about to say something reassuring, how it would be difficult to respond effectively since Tommy's attack was so unexpected—even social psychologists know a little about empathy—when Ruth bolted out of her seat, shouting. "That's enough, Larry, enough. Please stop it, now." She strode to where Larry was sitting and put a hand on his shoulder. He bowed his head and squeezed his eyes shut, trying to hold back the tears. Ruth stroked the back of his neck gently and Larry let go and began to cry quietly.

After a moment Larry stopped crying and regained his composure. Ruth continued to stand beside his chair as he told me about their experiences with Tommy following his attack on Ruth. He described how

Tommy's aggressive behavior had escalated, both at home and at school, including one incident where his third grade teacher called them in for a conference. A little girl who sat in front of Tommy had reported that he had threatened to gouge out her eyes if she didn't give her pencil to him. As he got older, his outbursts (and their fear) grew worse.

Larry also recounted their attempts to find help. At first, they sought advice and counseling from a succession of psychologists and psychiatrists in the community. While a few professionals, including Dr. Barker, seemed genuinely interested in trying to help, none of their efforts seemed to have a positive impact on Tommy's behavior. On several occasions his behavior actually deteriorated during treatment. To make matters worse many therapists made Ruth and Larry feel as if they were responsible for Tommy's problems. Sometimes the message was quite clear and explicit: They had not set firm limits for him as a young child, children always act out the conflicts that exist between their parents, therefore the Hammonds must have some unresolved marital problems. With other therapists, the guilt was induced more subtly and painfully, cloaked in a soft sheath of concerned questions and sympathetic gestures. Behind these expressions of concern lurked a sharp-edged judgment of attribution and blame which made them feel even worse.

After awhile, beaten down by frustration and guilt, they turned from the solo practitioners to agencies that supposedly had "programs" for children like Tommy. They went to mental health centers and family service agencies, made application to the special education program at the school and even tried to enroll Tommy in a day treatment program run by the child psychiatry division at the medical school. All to no avail. Either Tommy was not eligible for the program (the school psychologist told them his behavior didn't interfere with his educational functioning since he was receiving passing grades) or they had a long waiting list, or the agency decided his problems did not fall under their jurisdiction and suggested the Hammonds try agency X or Y or Z.

After awhile Tommy's outbursts became more explosive. Ruth was afraid to be alone with him and Larry cringed when she called him at work, dreading that Tommy had done something awful at school. One rainy day in April, when Tommy was ten, the dreaded call actually came. A little boy who had recently transferred from another school made the mistake of teasing Tommy. Without any warning, Tommy attacked the boy, knocking him to the ground and clawing at his face. When the teacher, a wispy middle-aged woman, tried to intervene, Tommy kicked her in the leg and ran out of the building into the street, where the burly vice-principal managed to tackle him.

The little boy required eleven stitches to close a deep gash on his face and the teacher's bruised shin caused her to miss two days of school. Tommy was suspended for ten days, and the school agreed not to press charges against Tommy only after the Hammonds promised to place him in the local private psychiatric hospital.

"If I knew then what I know now," Larry said, "I would have skipped all of those extra steps—and expenses—and gone directly to court. Tommy stayed in the hospital for twenty-eight days. He was released on the day my insurance benefits ran out. When he came home he was no different from when he went in, except that he was mad at us for putting him in the hospital.

"In the next year, he was admitted to hospitals twice more, the second time to the state hospital because we had no more insurance and had just about depleted our savings paying for his treatment."

"And none of it helped him at all," Ruth said angrily. "The therapists did a good job of making us feel guilty, but that's about it."

Larry nodded in agreement. "The only decent advice we got was from a tough, old social worker at the state hospital. She took us aside after one of those frustrating treatment meetings in which everyone agreed that Tommy's problems were serious, but no one had any practical ideas about what to do, short of sending him off to a residential treatment center for a couple of years.

"Neither Ruth nor I was prepared for that. It wasn't that we weren't ready emotionally. We were so desperate at that point we would have taken him to Lourdes if someone told us it might help Tommy. No, it was the money. Even the least expensive treatment center cost fifty to sixty thousand a year, which was a bargain compared to the big name places. Because of my income, we weren't eligible for any public assistance and there was no way we could afford to pay that kind of money."

"What about the schools?" I asked. "They couldn't possibly deny that his problems weren't interfering with his education, especially since they suspended him from school."

Larry smiled at me wistfully and I immediately felt like a fool. "We requested help, even went through a due process hearing where our request for residential treatment tuition assistance was denied. The school system argued they could meet his needs in a self-contained special education class within the regular school. Apparently their lawyers knew more about the laws than our lawyer. We lost the appeal."

I thought about the irony of the school telling the Hammonds they needed to put Tommy in a psychiatric hospital while at the same time claiming his educational needs could be met within a regular school. I decided not to say anything about this paradox. The Hammonds certainly didn't need to be reminded of how unfair the system was. "You were saying something about a social worker at the state hospital," I said.

"Oh, yes," Larry said. "I lost my train of thought. Seems to happen a lot lately. This woman-I think her name was Handler or Horner—"

"Handler," Ruth interjected. "Her name was Joan Handler. I'll never forget her name . . . or that day."

"That's right, Joan Handler," Larry said. "She wasn't exactly a warm and fuzzy type. But she was a straight shooter. She told us we were wasting our time. Tommy wasn't going to get the help he needed at the state hospital and none of the other agencies was going to shell out the money needed to get him the treatment he needed. She told us there was only one way Tommy could get the kind of treatment he needed, but the price would be very high."

I was confused. "I thought you had exhausted all of your savings?"

"Not that kind of price," Larry said, twisting his mouth into a joyless grin.

Once again, Ruth's anger broke through. This time it was directed at her husband. "For God's sake, Larry, do you have to drag it out? You act like this is some kind of suspense story! Well, it's not. When you close the book, nothing changes. We're still stuck with our miserable life. And Tommy is in big trouble."

Larry's face turned red. For a second he looked as if he was going to respond, but instead he took a deep breath, expelled it through his closed lips and continued. I noticed that Ruth made no effort to tell her version of what had happened, and Larry didn't encourage her to improve on his performance.

"The county social service department had a special fund for seriously disturbed kids," Larry said in a monotone. "Kids like Tommy. They were able to purchase intensive residential treatment for these kids if it could be demonstrated that no other services were suitable. The only catch was that funding was limited and they had to establish priorities for who would receive these services. Because the money was provided by the state, their highest priority—in fact, their only priority—was that the money be used for children who were wards of the state."

"So Tommy wasn't eligible?" I asked.

"That was our first reaction, too," Larry responded. "But the social worker told us his problems were so serious that they might be willing to support placement in a residential treatment center if we were willing to give up custody of Tommy and allow the social services department to become his legal guardians."

"That's absurd," I blurted out, stepping out of my professional investigator fact-finding role. "How could they make you give up custody of your own son?"

This time Ruth responded. Her anger had been replaced by sadness, a deep chasm of sadness that threatened to swallow her voice if not her entire being. "They didn't force us," she said in little more than a whisper. I had to lean forward to hear her. The photo album was still open to the boy with the crooked smile and his doting parents. "They gave us a choice. We could keep our son and watch him continue to deteriorate, or we could give up custody of our only son so the state could put him a place that might be able to help him."

There was no need for me to ask which alternative they had chosen.

CHAPTER THREE

Mommy and Daddy say they love me. All the time. They tell me they love me. Why did they send me away? I don't want to be here. I want my room. I want my games. They said they loved me.

The Onondaga Department of Social Services is located in a twenty-story glass and brick county building on South State Street. The county office building, which houses some of the area's nastiest bureaucrats, also has a reputation for demonstrating its unfriendliness to customers in a more tangible manner. Shortly after construction was completed, bricks became dislodged from the upper stories of the building, smashing into the sidewalk. The exterior wall was eventually reconstructed but the building continued to evoke fear in those who approached it.

The receptionist did not look pleased to see me. As I approached her desk, she put aside the bottle of red polish and began to study her nails. When I said hello she stopped examining her fingers and looked up at me but did not reply. Her glare was one part impatience and two parts disdain. I wondered whether it had been a bad day at work or trouble at home that made her so sour. Maybe she was just an unpleasant person.

After a moment of trying to empathize with her, my tolerance ran out. I didn't care if the boss had yelled at her or her child had the chicken pox. I and the other taxpayers of Onondaga County were paying her good money to provide a service and she was sitting there giving me the evil eye. Even if the money we were paying her wasn't so good (a possibility that had crossed my mind) I wasn't about to take any guff from someone who worked for a system that made parents give up their children to the state in order to get help.

"I'm here to see Mrs. Stamwell. I would appreciate it if you would let her know that I'm waiting for her."

The receptionist nodded once, then picked up the telephone receiver and punched in some numbers on the console. She mumbled a few words to the person on the other end, waited a moment and hung up the receiver. "Mrs. Stamwell will see you now. Go through the door behind me. Fifth door on the left."

What a letdown. I had been prepared to go all the way: righteous indignation, threats of notifying my county legislator, leaping over the reception desk and kicking in the door to the office area. She probably knew who she was dealing with.

As I started down the corridor, I realized, too late, she hadn't even asked my name.

Mrs. Stamwell was a tall black woman whose military posture made her look even larger than she was. She had gray hair pulled back tightly into a thick bun and intense dark brown eyes that would have made the most recalcitrant child-support scofflaw cough up his last nickel just to escape her gaze.

"What can I do for you, this afternoon?" she asked, looking at my scruffy shoes.

"Lou DeSantis suggested I call you. I've been hired by a family with a child in the care of your department. Their son is in trouble and they've asked me to assist them. Lou thought you might be able to help me."

"How is Lieutenant DeSantis? Still taking night courses at University College?"

Lou DeSantis was a detective at the Syracuse Police Department with a penchant for self-improvement. More accurately, Angie, his wife, had a strong desire for Lou to enhance his intellectual and cultural capacity, and he complied, usually without much of a fuss. He had been a student in a social psychology course I taught in the evening division. One night he stayed after class to ask me to explain attribution theory—a subject I've never been too clear on myself.

We discovered we had a number of common interests, including minor league hockey, the writings of Sir Arthur Conan Doyle, and good Italian food. Lou invited me to dinner (after the final grades were handed in) and one helping of Angie's duck lasagna with porcini and truffles convinced me this was a relationship worth pursuing.

Fortunately neither of us was hung up on having to root for a winning team. We saw a lot of bad hockey, ate some great pasta, and became good friends.

Sometimes Lou asked me to suggest a reference for a paper he was writing. Occasionally I sought his advice on one of my moonlight investigation jobs. On balance, I got more than I gave.

After speaking to the Hammonds, I had invited Lou to have a beer with me and asked him how I could learn more about Tommy Hammond. I wanted to find out how the professionals saw him, how they viewed his problems, whether he was capable of killing someone. But I also wanted to know about the bizarre system that had made his parents give up their child in order to get help for him.

Lou didn't hesitate. He told me Ernestine Stamwell knew more about child services than all the other welfare and mental health professionals in the county put together.

"Lou is doing well," I said. "He's taking a class in Greek mythology this semester."

Mrs. Stamwell chuckled. "Knowing Lieutenant DeSantis, he's probably telling his fellow officers about the similarities between Sisyphus and the bureaucratic burdens today's law enforcement officers are forced to bear."

"Speaking of bureaucracy," I said, "what can you tell me about Tommy Hammond?"

Her smile immediately turned into a frown. "I'm sorry, Mr. Fenton, I can't tell you anything about a particular child without a release of information authorization."

"No problem," I said, pulling a folded piece of paper from my shirt pocket. "The Hammonds signed a release form giving me access to their son's records."

"I have to give you credit. You've done your homework. But I'm afraid you're going to be disappointed. The district attorney in Northampton, Massachusetts subpoenaed all of Tommy's records, including the file we kept in this office. They're probably going through it with a magnifying glass."

I hadn't counted on that. "You mean his own parents can't have access to his records?"

Mrs. Stamwell shook her head slowly.

"What the hell kind of system is this?" I asked. "First you make the Hammonds give up custody of their only child. Then you send him away to some godforsaken institution in the middle of nowhere. Now, when he's accused of a serious crime, you put up a big stone wall between the boy and his family."

Mrs. Stamwell waited patiently until I had finished. Her nostrils flared and her eyes remained fixed on mine. When she spoke, it was in a soft, quiet voice. "We're not proud of ourselves. We know the system isn't fair. It tears families apart; it yanks kids out of their homes and neighborhoods, and puts them in places where they're likely to learn how to be better deviants. But we don't make the rules and we don't decide how much money should be allocated to help kids like Tommy. Those decisions are made by governors and legislators and other officials elected by the good people of our state. The same people who don't want taxes raised but want to build more prisons and detention centers so we can get rid of all deviants and criminals."

I felt like a seventh grader listening to a lecture on how democracy works. "So what's your point?" I said. "I'm not asking you to let perverts and murderers run wild because they had unhappy childhoods. I'm trying to find out how Tommy Hammond got into such a messy situation. I'm trying to figure out how a fourteen year-old boy with some heavy duty emotional problems gets taken away from his family, put into a residential treatment center in Massachusetts and ends up being charged with murder. And his parents can't even speak to Tommy because *your* agency has custody of him."

"I hope it makes you feel better to have a convenient scapegoat, Mr. Fenton. It must be nice to see the world so clearly: good guys and bad guys. If only it were so simple."

I felt a little foolish under the gaze of her dark eyes. "Look, maybe I have oversimplified the situation. But it sure beats the alternative, which is to accept things as they are, to let everyone off the hook—all those elected officials and high ranking government officials and, yes, even people like you—because people really don't care what happens to

Tommy Hammond and his family as long as it doesn't happen in their back yard."

Mrs. Stamwell started to respond, but thought better of it. Instead she reached for a pen and wrote something on a note pad on her desk. Tearing off the top page, she handed it to me. "You probably don't believe this, but we really don't see things much differently. I'm probably a little more jaded by age and experience, but not to the point of paralysis. I no longer have faith in quick fixes or magic bullets but I sure as hell haven't given up my belief in hard work and persistence. I hope you don't become frustrated too easily. You're going to need a lot of patience and stamina."

If my brief encounter with the "system" was any indication of what lay ahead, we agreed with each other on at least one thing.

I decided to stop at the Public Safety Building, which was only a block from Ernestine Stamwell's office. Lou was at his desk, bent over a stack of papers. As I approached, he pushed aside the papers and gave me a big grin. Although Lou loves to read and discuss ideas, he dislikes writing and especially hates police paperwork. I had no doubt that he was glad to see me, but I was also fairly certain his warm greeting had more to do with the welcome distraction I was providing than my scintillating personality. I tried not to take it personally.

"Hey, Sherlock," Lou said, "catch any runaway egos lately?"

"Funny," I responded, "What do you know about Jerome Hannigan?"

"Other than the fact that he is an extremely successful attorney, probably has more money than some small countries and is feared almost as much as he is despised by our venerable district attorney, not much."

"Sounds like quite a guy."

"Very impressive, but not exactly Mr. Congeniality. Rumor has it that Hannigan once brought his daughter to small claims court to recover part of her allowance because she was buying objectionable music. The story's probably apocryphal but the portrayal is accurate. I was the testifying officer in a narcotics trial in which Hannigan was defending a small-time drug dealer. He tore apart the prosecution case like a little kid unwrapping a Christmas present. After the jury acquitted the dealer, the young assistant D.A. who was handling the case approached Hannigan. The young guy—he couldn't have been more than twenty-five—tells Hannigan how much he admires his work, how it was an honor to appear in the same court. The assistant D.A. goes on like this for a couple of minutes, all the while Hannigan is gathering up his papers and stuffing them into his Gucci briefcase, not even looking at the kid. Finally, Hannigan picks up his briefcase and asks the assistant D.A. if he's done. When he says yes, Hannigan proceeds to lay him out in lavender. He says he's considering giving his client back his fee because he didn't earn it, since the state just about served up the case on a silver platter. Then he tells the assistant D.A. that isn't the only refund that's in order. He advises the assistant D.A. to request a refund from the law school he attended because they either didn't give him an adequate education or they accepted him under false pretenses, knowing he didn't have the brains to tend bar, no less practice law."

"Jesus, what did the kid do?"

"First he turned a deep shade of purple. Then he apologized to Hannigan for his ineptness. I thought he was going to get down on his knees and grovel for forgiveness. Two weeks later he resigned from the D.A.'s office. Last I heard he was closing loans for one of the less reputable mortgage companies in town. Anyway, why the interest in Hannigan?"

"I'm not sure. I had a frustrating conversation with Ernestine Stamwell, frustrating for both of us, I think. When we were finished she handed me a slip of paper with Hannigan's name and phone number on it."

Lou smiled. "I told you she knows more about this business than anyone I know. I'm not sure why she gave you Hannigan's number, but I'll bet you kopeks to knishes Hannigan can open some doors for you."

I thought of the young assistant D.A. and wondered whether the doors would lead in or out. Being a "nontraditional" (translates to older) graduate student I was less than confident about my academic prowess. Experience is supposed to instill wisdom and confidence. In my case, the only thing it had done was to make me more aware of the many ways I could screw up.

Would the Syracuse University Graduate School actually give someone a refund?

Better yet, what about the Ablemann School of Private Sector Investigation? Did that prestigious educational institution have a statute of limitations on revoking certification earned through its correspondence division?

The small plaque next to the elevator read: *Jerome F. Hannigan, Esq., Attorney-at-Law, Fourth Floor.* The setting certainly didn't match his reputation. The small building on West Fayette Street was neither attractive nor opulent. In fact, it was somewhat seedy, even by my modest standards. Nestled between two warehouses, the narrow brick building reminded me of something from a Mike Hammer movie. The kind of building I might have been in if I had remained in my previous profession. But hardly suitable for an upscale attorney.

The elevator rose at a snail's pace to the fourth floor. There were only two offices: the upstate branch of the New York State Antique Dealers Guild and Hannigan's. At least the Guild seemed to be in the right place.

I was greeted by a slim woman in her late forties or early fifties who wore her brown hair in a neatly wrapped bun. She sat at a beautiful dark wood desk, trimmed with gold plate. Perhaps they had gotten a discount from their neighbors.

"Can I help you, sir?" the woman with the bun said. She had a soft, gentle voice that made me want to ask her for milk and cookies.

"I hope so. I'm Marty Fenton. I called earlier to ask whether I could see Mr. Hannigan for a few minutes."

"Oh yes, I remember. Your timing is perfect. Mr. Hannigan just returned from court and has a few minutes before his next appointment. If you'll excuse me, I'll tell him you are here."

As she was speaking to Hannigan on the intercom I started to perspire. I hadn't stretched the truth *too* far when I had called. The Hammonds *were* victims of the legal system and they *were* in desperate need of counsel, though maybe not in the conventional sense. I hoped that Hannigan had already devoured his quota of young, over-educated males.

The woman with the bun led me into a large office tastefully decorated in contemporary Southwestern decor. The desert colors were a stark contrast to the rest of the building. The large red and black R.C. Gorman painting that hung behind the lawyer's desk made me think of the Sangre de Cristo Mountains outside of Santa Fe, a far cry from West Fayette Street.

When Jerome Hannigan rose from his desk, I expected a turquoise bolo and alligator boots. Instead, he wore a light gray silk suit with a muted burgundy and blue floral tie. The only concession to his Southwestern office decor was the large silver buckle on his belt. He was a tall, athletic man with stylishly long silver hair and a deep tan that probably hadn't come from a salon. His pale gray eyes focused intently on me from behind silver wire rimmed glasses. He shook my hand firmly and motioned me to sit on a mauve sofa while he sat in a high backed wooden chair with a leather seat across from me.

"What kind of problems are you having with our less-than-perfect system of justice?" he asked in a resonant voice that would have assured him a spot on Pavarotti's road team.

I've never been a good liar. "Uh, it's not exactly my problem."

The pale gray eyes bore into me. I sought relief from the top of my shoes. "Whose problem are we discussing, Mr. Fenton?"

I spoke quickly, hoping to convince him of the urgency of my mission— and to deter him from delivering one of his lethal assistant D.A. retorts. I told him about Ruth and Larry Hammond, their problems with Tommy, the obstacles they ran into trying to find help for him. I explained how they had been forced to give up custody of their son in order to place him in the residential treatment center in Massachusetts. Finally I raced through the story of the youngster being killed at the treatment center, the allegations against Tommy, and the Hammonds' inability to speak to Tommy or get any information because they no longer had custody.

Hannigan sat quietly as I recounted the background that led me to seek his help. When I finished, he removed his glasses and rubbed his eyes. Then he leaned forward and said, "I ought to throw your ass out of my office right now. You misrepresented yourself to get access to me. You told me you had a problem with the legal system when it wasn't your problem at all. Then you come in here and try to snow me with this sad story without even offering an apology."

"Would it help if I apologized now?"

"No, it wouldn't. Not a bit. Who the hell are you anyway?"

"I . . . I, uh . . . work part time as a private investigator. I'm working for the Hammonds."

"I sure hope you don't rely on your part-time profession to put bread on the table. If your clients pay you for what you're worth, you won't need to worry about the IRS. You won't make enough to need to file a tax return."

I decided to treat his remark about my work as rhetorical. I had no desire to find out what choice comments he would make about my other career. "I'm sorry," I said, realizing as I spoke that Hannigan had just told me not to apologize. "I didn't mean to deceive you. But I didn't really have much choice. My clients are desperate. Their son has been accused of murder. They can't even talk to him. Nobody's giving them or me any information. What the hell do you expect me to do? I know you're a busy man. When your secretary asked me why I wanted to see you I didn't pay much attention to personal pronouns. Maybe I cut a few corners, but I wasn't trying to mislead you. If you want to throw me out of your office, go ahead. But let's stop playing head games. This isn't helping anyone, least of all my clients."

In psychology they call it a counter-phobic response, tackling head on what you're most afraid of. On the streets of Teaneck, New Jersey, where I grew up, my Jewish friends called it chutzpah.

I braced myself for Hannigan's response.

"Why did you come to me?" he asked. "Who gave you my name?"

Not exactly what I expected from the man eater. Was he lulling me into a false sense of complacency? "One of the supervisors from the Department of Social Services. Ernestine Stamwell."

Hannigan closed his eyes and put his hand to his forehead. "Jesus, why didn't you say something earlier? It would have saved both of us a lot of aggravation."

I was tempted to say he hadn't asked me, but thought better of it. "Would it have made a difference?" I replied instead.

"Hell yes. Ernie Stamwell is one special lady. I take her referrals very seriously."

I didn't get it. Here was this extraordinarily successful, arrogant attorney, a man who blew away other lawyers with a flick of his tongue, doing a 180 degree turn at the mention of a social worker's name. What was it about this welfare bureaucrat that evoked such a strong response from Hannigan? Did she have something on him? A secret he didn't want revealed, an indiscreet act he had committed? A legal short cut he had taken? Whatever she had, I was grateful she had chosen to use it on behalf of the Hammonds. In spite of my curiosity, I wasn't about to risk provoking Hannigan's ire by asking him why she was special.

"Does this mean you're going to help . . . the Hammonds?" I asked.

"Don't get too cocky, Fenton. What I'm willing to do is talk to your clients. If they give me something to work with, I'll make some calls, see if I can open some doors. What I need for you to do is to contact these people, let them know I'm willing to speak with them. Just make sure you don't oversell what I can do. I'm not promising anything at this point. If they want to pursue this, have them call me at this number." He took a business card from his billfold and handed it to me. I glanced at the card. Gold embossed lettering. "And Fenton, the invitation to call doesn't extend to you. The only good thing I can say about you is that you didn't let me know who your clients are. At least you retained something they taught you in whatever second-rate private-eye school you attended."

Not fair. Ablemann's School was certified by the National Association of Private Investigators. Somehow I didn't think Hannigan would be impressed by this credential. I decided to cut my losses and exit graciously. I tucked the business card in my shirt pocket, thanked him for his willingness to speak with my clients, and quickly left the bright Southwestern office before Hannigan could unleash another opinion.

I called the Hammonds from a pay phone and told them about my conversations with Ernestine Stamwell and Jerome Hannigan. With Ruth on one phone and Larry on the other, I felt like the proverbial ping pong ball as they argued about the intentions of the social worker and the lawyer. Ruth was worried that Mrs. Stamwell would mistake their inquiry for an attack on her department and might try to terminate funding for Tommy. Larry thought she was mistaken. He saw Mrs. Stamwell as a hard working social worker who was embarrassed by the bureaucracy she worked for and was trying to steer them toward help. But Larry didn't trust Hannigan. He was convinced the lawyer only wanted to lure them into a high-fee arrangement to represent Tommy. Ruth disagreed. She saw Hannigan as their last hope . . . their only hope.

It was painful to hear the Hammonds bickering. I thought of the photo album in Ruth Hammond's lap and the happy pictures of Tommy and his parents. How different those photographs would look if they were taken now. The ordeal with Tommy had not only left them poor and disillusioned. It had also sapped their emotional strength. Both of them were beaten and defeated and seemed to have only enough energy to strike out at the nearest target, to pick at each other's open wounds. And how about Tommy? I couldn't imagine what this experience had done to him.

After a moment they stopped arguing and agreed to call Hannigan. I told them I thought that was a good decision and promised to check in with them the following afternoon. They thanked me for responding so quickly and wished me a good evening. I didn't know what kind of evening I would have, but guessed it would be better than theirs.

On the way to my car I considered my options. There was nothing more I could do about Tommy Hammond. That would have to wait until Jerome Hannigan did his thing. There was always my thesis. I owed Professor Singleton a chapter and it wasn't going to write itself. Unfortunately I couldn't muster much enthusiasm for scholarly endeavor. Besides, Singleton was responsible for getting me involved with the Hammonds. Certainly he wouldn't begrudge me a little respite from the intensity of my intellectual pursuits. And if he did . . . well that was too bad.

Which left me only one viable option.

CHAPTER FOUR

*The doctor keeps looking at me. She asks me why I hurt the
boy. I tell her I didn't. I just wanted him to go away. He was
so close and he said bad things to me. I told him to leave me
alone but he didn't. It wasn't my fault.*

Ollie almost never went directly home after work. Three evenings
she went to Earl's gym to work out. Earl's was not your typical
Yuppie fitness center with bright lights, designer carpets,
polished machines and a health-drink bar. The motif at Earl's was simpler:
large iron barbells, a few frayed benches and an old soda machine. The
Spartan environment at Earl's was well suited for Ollie's purpose. She
didn't come to the gym to show off her spandex tights and sip papaya
juice. When I asked about watching her work out, she made it clear to
me that I would be at risk of serious bodily harm if I ever crossed the
threshold of Earl's gym when she was there.

It was not a threat I wished to challenge.

Fortunately this was not one of her nights at Earl's. The other two
nights she went to the university sculpture studio where she focused her
energy on creating large, abstract art forms. Unlike Earl's gym and the
bodybuilding arena, this place was not out of bounds for me. Ollie was
not self-conscious about me watching her sculpt and, in fact, sometimes
asked me to keep her company while she worked. Lately however, she
hadn't invited me to the studio.

The wood sculpture studio was housed in the red brick panel visual
arts building on the edge of campus. As always, it was filled with students
of all ages cutting, chiseling, and sanding their works of art. Ollie was in
her usual spot in a rear corner of the studio. She was bent over a large

teak figure, gouging out chunks of wood with a thick steel instrument. Like the other sculptors, she wore safety glasses.

Ollie was engrossed in her work and didn't see me right away. I stood quietly and watched how easily she manipulated the chisel. As always, I was impressed by her strength and agility. Not long ago, while I was working on another case, she had come to my rescue when some bad guys had threatened to do me bodily harm, and I had developed a real appreciation for her physical prowess.

But there was much more to Ollie than her physical prowess. She was an assertive woman who retained her femininity while demonstrating, in countless ways, that she could hold her own with members of the male gender, intellectually and socially as well as physically.

I admired her independence, though I had to admit it troubled me more than a little, especially since my long-standing aversion to commitment in male-female relationships had weakened considerably as my feelings for Ollie grew. I had always been the one to shy away from "getting serious." Now the roles were reversed. I was ready to make a long-term commitment, but Ollie was content to enjoy our time together without worrying about the future.

This was not the only irony. In what seemed to be an especially cruel twist of fate, now that we had finally begun to communicate honestly, the things we had always enjoyed together, the everyday pleasures of being in each other's company, had begun to lose their sparkle.

Just as I had reached the point where I no longer felt the need to constantly push for a commitment, and Ollie began to shed some of her protective armor, we started to lose interest in the things that had always sustained us. We no longer scanned the weekend section of the newspaper to see which ethnic festival was being held or where our favorite jazz trio was playing. We didn't grab our toboggan and drive to Green Lakes every time there was a decent snowfall—which occurred frequently in Syracuse. Even our sexual relationship, which had been incredible, was less spontaneous and intense.

As I watched Ollie shape the wooden form I was aware of another aspect of her personality, one that I had not noticed—or she had not revealed—until recently. Beneath Ollie's strength and competence, her independence and tenacity, there was a vulnerable woman who no longer wanted to keep the world out, but was not sure how to let one person in.

I wanted to take Ollie in my arms, to hold her and tell her it was okay, that everything would be alright. But I couldn't. Not from lack of desire, but because I wasn't really certain it was going to be alright.

Ollie looked up and smiled as I approached her. "Hey, stranger, I thought you'd gone to Russia to take drooling lessons from Pavlov's dogs."

This was new. Ollie had a great sense of humor. She had always been able to catch me off guard with one of her dry, witty remarks. She was as good as anyone I knew at using humor to remind me of my many personal quirks. But in the past her jokes had always been gentle and lighthearted. Now her humor had a biting, hostile edge that made me uncomfortable.

"I couldn't get my visa in time," I responded feebly. "Maybe next month." This conversation was starting off badly. I didn't like her remark and I thought even less of my response. Why couldn't I be more direct with Ollie?

"I'm surprised to see you, Marty. I thought you were working feverishly on your dissertation." Not nearly as nasty.

"I picked up a new case and thought I'd stop by to see you on my way home."

"Do you really have time for a case?" she asked.

Real smooth, Fenton, I thought. I was rapidly sliding out of the pan into the fire. Ollie had gotten me out of a couple of jams on my last case, at some risk to herself. At one point she had been abducted at gunpoint by some nasty people who didn't want me to continue snooping around. If it hadn't been for her quick reflexes neither of us would have been standing in the middle of the sculpture studio engaged in this convoluted attempt to communicate with each other.

To say that Ollie was ambivalent about my moonlighting activities would be a gross understatement.

"Actually Professor Singleton asked me to take the job. Besides, I can use the money."

"There are other ways to earn money," Ollie said, "and if you're really concerned about personal finances the best thing you could do is finish your dissertation so you can get a real job." She jabbed her chisel into the wood and began to gouge.

My tolerance for oblique conversation is pretty high, but even I have limits. "Look, Ollie, I really came to talk to you about what's happening with us. I thought we had worked things out after we found Fred Majorski. I realized I had been coming on pretty strong, that my intensity had more to do with my own issues than you. I think I've been doing a pretty good job of not pressuring you. But you seem to be even more upset with me than you were before."

Ollie put down her carving tool and turned to me. She removed her goggles. Her eyes were red. "I'm sorry. It's not you, Marty. It's just . . ." She took a deep breath and exhaled. "Can we get out of here?" she asked.

"Sure. No problem." I hadn't seen Ollie like this before. She almost always seemed to be in complete control of herself. On a few occasions, when I said something to make her angry, she had lashed out at me—with words only, fortunately. But I had never seen her like this. It made me nervous.

"Where do you want to go?" I asked.

"I don't care," she said softly.

I helped her put on her jacket and we left the studio. The temperature had dropped and, even though it was early April, the cold, damp air signaled that snow was on its way. I had become fairly well acclimated to the harsh winters of central New York but was not certain I would ever become accustomed to the April and May snow squalls.

I looked at Ollie. She was shivering. I suggested we take my car, which was parked a few feet away, and come back later for her car. She nodded.

I considered taking Ollie to my apartment, but there was something about going to my place that didn't feel right. I decided not to go to her place for the same reason.

Ollie was not the only one whose behavior was out of character that night.

As we drove along Comstock Avenue I tried to think of a good place to go, someplace quiet where we could talk. Most of our usual hangouts were too crowded and noisy. Thinking of these places made me hungry. I was about to ask Ollie if she wanted to get something to eat, but before I could say anything she said, "Could you take me back to my car? I don't feel well and I'd like to go home."

"But I thought you wanted to talk?" I said, surprised by her change of mind.

"I thought I did but I guess I'm not ready."

Ready for what? Now I was really nervous. "What's going on, Ollie? I know you well enough to know that something's bothering you. Yet every time I try to speak with you, I feel like I'm being brushed aside. Back at the studio you said it's not me, but it's getting harder for me to believe that."

Ollie fidgeted with her hands in her lap. "I wish I could be more clear about it myself," she said. "I know you've been working hard at not being so caught up in how our relationship is going. I appreciate your willingness to back off. I know it isn't easy. But even though you're doing what I asked you to do, I'm still feeling uncomfortable and I don't know why. I got what I wanted and now I'm more uncomfortable than I was before."

I was silent and concentrated on driving.

By this time we were on the outskirts of the city and I had no idea where we were going. "Can we go back to my car?" Ollie asked, sounding even more despondent.

I had exhausted my repertoire of clever responses so I turned around and drove back to the studio. Neither of us spoke on the return trip. Pulling in next to Ollie's Volkswagen, I shifted into neutral and put on the emergency brake. "Can't we talk about this?" I asked, not liking the whining tone of my voice.

"Not now," Ollie responded. "I need some time by myself to sort this out. I know you mean well, Marty, but when we talk I feel like you're looking for me to give you the right answer, to say something that will make everything okay . . . I don't know if I can do that. And the pressure I feel certainly doesn't help me think clearly."

"I'm sorry," I said lamely.

"It's not your fault. I know you care about me and want things to work out for us. I also know you've been trying to focus on what's happening with us now and not dwell on the future, and I appreciate that. I really do. Unfortunately I'm not able to bring much to our relationship right now. But that's just the way it is and you can't do anything about it."

I was a slow learner, but I had managed to figure out a few things about Ollie early in our relationship. Lesson number one was when she made up her mind there was nothing anyone could do to make her change it.

As I watched Ollie back out of the parking space, I turned my mind to less complicated subjects. I thought about what I would have for dinner and how I hadn't done my laundry for more than a week. I wondered why I hadn't received the latest copy of *Puzzle Monthly* and then remembered I had forgotten to renew my subscription.

The last thing I thought about before I sank into a warm vat of self-pity was Jerome Hannigan.

I wondered how he would have handled the situation with Ollie. I didn't know what he would do to break the impasse, but I was fairly certain he wouldn't resort to some pseudo- Freudian ploy to jog her memory.

I decided to forgo my laundry in favor of getting something to eat and working on my thesis. Putting on a shirt I had worn before didn't bother me nearly as much as having my stomach growl. And the guilt I would feel if I let down my advisor again was certainly worse than any self-consciousness I would feel being seen in a wrinkled shirt. Dressing for success was not one of my strong points.

I wolfed down a club sandwich at the Varsity, and then walked two short blocks to the library. Bird Library is a square gray structure that sits on the end of Walnut Avenue, on the edge of the academic quad, standing sentry over the fraternity and sorority houses that line the wide avenue to the north.

Rumor had it that when the library was built in the seventies, its designers did not take into account the enormous weight of the books. To avoid the embarrassment of having the building sink into the ground, the contractor reinforced the foundation. I have always been skeptical about the credibility of this story, especially since I have heard similar accounts about other college libraries. But my experience with the construction industry made me reluctant to dismiss the possibility that this engineering blunder actually occurred.

As I entered the large foyer of the library I felt myself relax. I love spending time in libraries. Surrounded by such a wealth of knowledge I have difficulty deciding what I want to read: the classics of literature, the wonders of science, or the trivia of popular culture. I wander through the stacks, scanning the shelves until I find something interesting. Then I pluck the volume I want from the shelf and hurry to a cubicle where I open the book and lock my eyes onto the clear black print. Once I start to read I won't put down the book until I am finished. I lose track of time and on occasion have even ignored my stomach's cries of hunger and skipped a meal.

I have always considered my stack-searching inclination a positive attribute. Ollie, on the other hand, views my exploratory tendencies as nothing more than another way to avoid working on my thesis. In truth, neither of us is completely wrong.

That night I was determined to do some serious work on my results section. How difficult could it be? I just had to describe the statistical procedures I used to analyze my data, report the results and indicate whether they were statistically significant.

I opened my thesis folder, ready to plunge in. Then I remembered. Just a small detail, but an important one nonetheless.

I had neglected to go to the computer lab to run my stats. I was so preoccupied with overcoming the barriers that kept me from finding out what was happening with Tommy Hammond—as well as Ollie—that I had forgotten about doing my data analysis. Maybe I had a learning disability. Or maybe Freud was right when he said we do only what we really want to do.

Of course I could still trot over to the computer lab. It was only a few blocks away. Or I could spend some time learning about the strange mental health system that made a child's parents give up custody in order to receive help.

It did not take me long to decide.

The advances that have been made in library research technology since I was an undergraduate are wonderful. No longer do I have to thumb through tightly packed stacks of catalogue cards or pull from shelves multiple volumes of periodical indexes. With a few strokes on the keyboard I can bring up on the screen neatly ordered lists of reference sources, organized by author, title, subject, or keyword. Without leaving my chair I can then call up an abstract of any article that looks promising to see whether it is worth pursuing.

The best part is that even after I locate an article or book I want, I don't have to walk up and down the musty aisles of the stacks searching for the right volume. With my exalted status as a graduate student I am granted the privilege of punching in a code on the computer that mobilizes a crack team of undergraduate work-study students. As soon as they receive my signal, the team descends upon the stacks, retrieves the reference materials I want, makes copies of the pertinent articles or chapters, and delivers them post-haste to the reference desk where I can pick them up or have them sent to my office through campus mail.

To be totally candid, these privileges are not afforded to all graduate students. The fact that my research overlaps with Professor Singleton's interests, prompting him to put me on the research grant he got from the National Institute of Mental Health, may have something to do with my access to this special service.

I walked up a flight of stairs to the next level. There was a single computer terminal in a small alcove hidden behind the section where the oversized books were shelved. Most students did not know it was there. It was almost never used.

No one was sitting at the terminal. On the screen was a list of journal article titles under the heading, "Obsessive-Compulsive Disorders in Children."

Maybe it wasn't a coincidence. Maybe it was fate. What was I saying? Here I was, a graduate student in psychology, engaged in the systematic application of scientific methods to understand human behavior. And what was I doing? Reaching for straws. Relying on the well-known scientific principle of "fate" to explain why the computer terminal I happened to select was displaying a reference that not only coincided with my field of study, but may also have been relevant to the case I had just accepted.

Get a grip, Fenton. You're really out of control.

I cleared the screen and typed in *K* for "keyword" and then *Child mental health*. I tapped the *Enter* key and waited as the computer searched its files. In less than a minute a summary of the search appeared on the screen. The computer had found 7,462 references under the key words *Child mental health*. Too many items. It would take hours to run through the list.

I tried several other keyword combinations but they either produced too many items or brought up my least favorite message: *no references found under this heading*. Just as I was about to give up, I found what I was looking for. When I typed in *services for children, problems,* the computer produced fifty-three references, a manageable list.

The references were arranged in reverse chronological order, with each year organized alphabetically by title. I didn't find anything interesting that had been published in the last few years, but when I reached 1992 I found a reference entitled *Requiring parents of children with emotional disturbance to transfer custody in order to obtain services: Practices and problems.* I jotted down the name of the journal and pertinent information about the article, and set out for the periodical section.

When I began my graduate studies I was intimidated by the library. The computer catalogue system baffled me. Each time I tried to use it the cursor seemed to lock up. Not being a person who pays much attention to written directions, it took me a few weeks to figure out that I could solve that problem with a couple of strokes on the keyboard.

The stack system also frustrated me. The library in my undergraduate college was small and compact. If they had a volume I was looking for— and they didn't have many—it was easy to find. But Bird Library, with its nearly three million volumes, was a different story. There were endless rows of books and even though the catalogue numbers were printed clearly at the beginning of each aisle, I would invariably walk past the book I was looking for several times before I found it.

That is, if it hadn't been checked out or sent to the bindery or improperly shelved or simply vanished.

The more frustrated I became with the huge library, the more determined I was to figure out how to make it work for me. I wasn't going to let this so-called repository of knowledge, with its technological sophistication and bureaucratic inefficiency, lock me out. I've always felt libraries were special places. You could go anywhere in the world without leaving the building; contemplate the ideas of the great philosophers or explore the wonders of science by simply plucking a book from a shelf. I'd be damned if I was going to let this system deny me all of that wonderful knowledge. It was not merely a question of figuring out how to use the computer catalogue or how to locate a book on a shelf. It had become a personal challenge for me. I was going to master the Bird Library System, even it I had to spend every waking moment in that ugly building.

Fortunately for me, it was not a formidable challenge. After a few weeks I figured out how to use the computer, learned how to find my way around the stacks, and made friends with a few members of the staff who had been there long enough to know how to retrieve books I couldn't locate through conventional channels.

Bird Library, which had given me nothing but aggravation and frustration, now became a great source of stimulation and gratification as I spent hours perusing its cloth-covered books and spooling the microfilm machines.

I don't know if my mother is right when she says that I turn ordinary problems into fascinating puzzles which then become all-consuming obsessions. My mother may be correct about my reluctance to give up something once I have started —my words, not hers—but I don't think it's a perfect theory. After all, if I was so tenacious about seeing a project through to completion, why was I having so much trouble finishing up my thesis?

Good question, huh?

The article on custody transfer had a lot of technical terms. After reading it for a second time I thought I understood it. The authors had conducted a national survey and found that nearly two-thirds of all states still made parents give up custody if they wanted the agencies to pay for the special services their kids needed. Most of the reasons given for continuing this barbaric practice were pretty pathetic: it was a federal requirement, the parents might undermine the treatment program, the program wasn't intended for kids who were emotionally disturbed. The authors of the article were more generous than I would have been. They concluded that the real problem was that these agencies really weren't geared up to work with families who had children with serious emotional problems. Many of the staff still believed the only reason kids had emotional disorders was that their parents mistreated them. The authors pointed out that there was a growing body of research evidence supporting the theory that many children were genetically predisposed to mental illness.

For professionals who knew better, there didn't seem to be many good options. There wasn't enough money to treat all the kids who needed help. With the shortage of resources, parents were often forced to turn to funding sources that were originally intended for children who had been abused, a situation in which it was reasonable for the state to take charge, at least temporarily.

To make matters worse, the limited funds available were being used to send kids to large residential facilities, which were not only expensive but also tore these children away from their families, unlike programs that treated children at home and in the community.

For me, it boiled down to one thing: The United States of America, the most powerful country in the world, didn't care enough about these kids and families to do the right thing. We can launch a cruise missile and drop it into the back yard of a hostile dictator a thousand miles away, but we can't treat a vulnerable child without severing the relationship between a son and his parents. So Ruth and Larry Hammond had been forced to give up custody of their only child in order to get help for him. Now this boy was being held in a small city two hundred miles from his home, accused of killing another youngster . And his parents didn't even know where he was.

I closed the book and placed it on the reshelving cart. Not a very fruitful evening. I had learned a little more about the child mental health system but I didn't feel any wiser. As for my thesis . . . it would have to wait for another day

CHAPTER FIVE

Where is Bernard? I don't like it here. I want my bed and my blanket and my monkey. I should have my snack. I always have my snack before I go to bed. It's not fair. They should give me my snack. They should take me back to my room. I don't like them. They're not nice. They're going to hurt me. I'm scared.

I awoke to the sound of rain pinging on my window. I had hoped to get an early start on my data analysis before fatigue and rumination wore down my resolve. When I first looked out the window and saw how dark the sky was, I was excited. I would grab a bagel and a quick cup of coffee and hurry to the computer lab before all of the PCs were taken. A few hours of steady crunching and all of the data would be analyzed. Then all I would have to do is write up the results and explain my findings.

Maybe if I hadn't glanced at the clock radio I would have followed through on my plan. But when I saw that it was 10:15 A.M. and just another gray Syracuse day, my determination dissolved.

After a warm shower and a bowl of Cheerios—the bagels were too stale, even for me—I called the Hammonds' home to find out if they had heard from Jerome Hannigan. Ruth answered the phone and, for the first time since I met her, sounded as if she might complete a sentence without breaking into tears. In fact, she seemed almost cheerful as she told me that Hannigan had just called with some good news. He had convinced the family court judge that it was not in Tommy's or his parents' best interest to keep them in the dark about what was happening with him. The judge had issued an order allowing the Hammonds or their designee to speak to the staff of the residential treatment center as well as the county attorney handling Tommy's case. He also gave them permission to visit Tommy in the juvenile detention center.

The Hammonds had asked Hannigan to represent Tommy, but he told them he was in the middle of a very complicated case and wouldn't be able to leave Syracuse for several weeks. He did, however, give them the name of a colleague in Northampton, which was only ten miles away from the town where Tommy was being held.

The Hammonds decided to wait until the weekend to visit Tommy. Larry had an important presentation to make the next day and Ruth felt she needed a couple of days to compose herself. She was afraid that if Tommy saw her in such an emotional state he might become even more disturbed. I thought it was odd that they didn't want to see Tommy immediately but then I didn't really know what it was like to be in their situation. I had difficulty knowing how to respond when Ollie became angry with me. I couldn't begin to fathom what it would be like to have your own child turn against you for no apparent reason, watch him withdraw from you and the rest of the world, and not only feel helpless to do anything for him, but be told the only way he can receive assistance is if you give him up to some bureaucratic system.

Larry asked if I would be willing to serve as their designee. They wanted me to meet with the county attorney and their lawyer as well as to visit the treatment center. I told them I would pick up the judge's order after my afternoon class. With any luck I would be able to reach the lawyers and the treatment center and set up appointments for the next day. If I left early I could be in western Massachusetts before noon.

As soon as I hung up I regretted my decision to wait until after class to get the judge's orders. My one o'clock class was with Professor Singleton. He would undoubtedly ask if my results section was on schedule and I would be forced to swallow hard and tell him it was going to be late. I had learned the hard way not to give excuses to Professor Singleton. He had an uncanny ability to engage in prolonged explorations of how students were feeling about their grandmother's death or the broken furnace or whatever alleged calamity had prevented them from completing their work on time. Though his tone was usually sympathetic, the student's suffering was always intense. Much better to get it over quickly than to prolong the agony.

If I had chosen to "get on the case" immediately I would have avoided, or at least postponed, the humiliation of telling Singleton I had once again failed to produce the results section of my thesis.

I was able to reach the county attorney and the residential treatment center but not the lawyer Hannigan had recommended. I suffered through Singleton's class—he waited until the end of class to ask about my progress—and stopped by the courthouse to pick up the judge's order. After enduring an intensive interrogation by a clerk who made F. Lee Bailey look like a creampuff, I was able to convince her I was representing the Hammonds and she grudgingly gave me the court order.

My visit to the courthouse had rekindled my frustration with the children's service system. Nothing came easily. There were always rules to follow, forms to fill out, and red tape to untangle. All of the special requirements were supposed to be in the best interest of the child, but I had my doubts. The only people who seemed to benefit from these inane procedures were the bureaucrats whose job security was significantly enhanced by the workload created by the special requirements.

My visit to the courthouse left me with a lot of toxic feelings. I decided to channel my energy productively rather than risk being held in contempt for the input I was inclined to provide the court personnel. I drove back to campus and went to the computer lab. This time I remembered to bring my data.

The computer lab is a large windowless room. It is brightly lit by an ample bank of recessed fluorescent lights, and has a peculiar odor that I attribute to emissions from the burning brain cells of students frustrated with the computers' supposedly user-friendly software programs. The lab is open seven days a week, twenty-four hours a day, but every time I went there it felt like the middle of the night.

Along one side of the room was a row of printers: laser printers for finished copies of papers and reports, and noisy dot matrix machines for draft work and statistical printouts. The clatter of the printers and the quieter but equally annoying sound of keyboard stroking almost always gave me a headache. On a bad day I was ready for Tylenol in forty-five minutes.

As soon as I entered the lab I noticed the difference. The printers weren't whirring, the keyboards weren't clicking. In fact, there was no noise at all. One lone student sat in front of a PC at the far end of the room reading. The screen was lit up but his attention was turned to a large paperback book.

I took the silence to be a good omen and quickly got to work. Selecting a Hewlett-Packard near the door, I pulled out my data disk, inserted it into the slot, and loaded the data into the computer. Then I activated the SAS statistical package and began to crunch my data. Just as I was about to complete my first series of tests I heard the door open. I was so engrossed in my work that I didn't look up until I sensed that someone was standing next to me. When I turned to see who it was, I was so surprised I actually gasped.

Ollie stood with arms crossed in front of her, grinning like a Cheshire cat.

"Wha . . . what are you doing here?" I stammered.

"Enjoying the sight of your mouth hanging open," she responded.

"No, I mean how come you came here? How did you know I was here? And before you say anything, stop looking at me like that."

Ollie tried to suppress her smile but didn't succeed completely. "I called your apartment and got no answer. Then I went to the library because I remembered you owed Singleton a chapter. When I didn't find you in the stacks I figured you might be here. You're not the only detective on campus, you know." Ollie paused and took a deep breath. She was no longer smiling. "I didn't like the way things ended last night."

"Neither did I. It was pretty frustrating. I really wanted to talk with you, but—"

"I know. I wasn't feeling very communicative. As I said last night, I just wasn't ready for that conversation."

"And now?" I asked cautiously.

Ollie furrowed her brow and looked down at me. Then she smiled, "Right now I would like to buy you a cup of coffee and split a large slice of chocolate cake. If you need some time to finish up here I brought a book to read. Mostly I don't want to hassle about our relationship. I'd like to have a nice relaxing time together, if that's okay with you."

It was definitely okay with me. I downloaded the SAS program, inserted my data disk, and ran the first set of my statistical tests. To my delight I didn't make any mistakes. Even better, my first two hypotheses turned out to be statistically significant in the predicted direction. To a research psychologist that was on the same level as winning the lottery or getting a date with someone you've had a crush on for a long time.

I decided to quit while I was ahead. I gathered up my papers, Ollie closed her book and we left the computer lab. I was excited about her unexpected visit but still unsure about why she had come. I hoped her offer to buy me coffee and cake wasn't intended to buffer bad news.

"So where would you like to go?" I asked.

"I don't know. I was thinking of the diner on Erie Boulevard. That sound okay to you?"

I nodded, grateful not to have to make a decision.

We took her VW which was older and less comfortable than my Honda, but had recently been more reliable. Contrary to popular opinion, Japanese cars sometimes break down. Of course the fact that my Accord has over two hundred thousand miles on the odometer may have had some bearing on its current performance.

The diner, which was usually filled with customers, was almost empty. We managed to find a booth in the back. No one else was sitting in that section. We placed our order with a friendly waitress who engaged us in the favorite local pastime: talking about the weather. After she left, Ollie cleared her throat, "Last night must have seemed pretty strange to you, huh?"

My first impulse was to tell her the night had seemed normal; she was the one that seemed strange! But I decided that such a comment wouldn't advance our conversation. "I didn't feel good about it," I said instead. "You seemed to be upset but I couldn't figure out what was bothering you."

Ollie smiled. "You psychology students are all alike, trying to analyze every little statement or gesture. Who was it that said 'sometimes a cigar is just a cigar'?"

Her phallic reference did not make me feel more comfortable. "Come on, Ollie. That's not fair. I wasn't trying to find any deep psychological meaning. I don't like to see you upset; especially when I think it has something to do with me."

"I'm sorry," Ollie said, reaching over to pat my arm. "I'm having trouble with this. I'll try to be more focused."

"Apology accepted, and it was Freud."

"What?"

"Sigmund Freud. He's the one who said 'sometimes a cigar is just a cigar.'"

Ollie shook her head, and then took a sip of coffee. "Lately I've found myself feeling angry at you. Most of the time it doesn't seem to have anything to do with what you're doing at the time or even what's going on between us. We could be sitting together talking like we are now and I'll suddenly become irritated with you. Right now, in fact, the way you're fidgeting with your coffee cup bothers me. Another time I became annoyed because you were speaking too loudly even though your tone was the same as it always is. I know it doesn't make sense, but sometimes I get so mad at these little things that I just want to smack you."

"Thank goodness for self-restraint," I muttered, removing my hands from the coffee cup.

"I'm serious, Marty. I don't like feeling this way. I'm usually in touch with my feelings. When I'm angry I know why. But this is different. Something's going on with me and I don't understand it."

Ollie looked down at her plate. She looked like she was on the verge of tears and I didn't know what to do. I wanted to comfort her but was afraid I would make her even angrier. I also was more than a little curious about why she was reacting this way to me. For once I wished I knew something about the people side of psychology. "Is there something I can do?" I asked hesitantly.

Ollie looked up at me and forced a smile. "I know this is hard for you and I wish I could tell you why I'm reacting this way. I honestly don't know if it's something about our relationship that's bothering me or if I'm just venting my anger on you because you're a safe target. The only thing I'm certain about is that things are just going to get worse unless I deal with this."

"Do you think it would be helpful for us to talk about it?"

"I don't know. I really don't. I guess it would be good for us to try, but I can't make any promises."

"That's okay. I understand this is hard for you. Why don't we give it a try?" Jesus, I was beginning to sound like a clinician.

"Okay, but I'm not really up for it tonight. Could we talk tomorrow?"

Bob Cohen

Just my luck. Ollie finally decides to open up and I'm leaving town. "Uh, do you think it could wait for a few days?" Ollie furrowed her brow. I couldn't tell if she was disappointed or just puzzled, though my ego hoped it was disappointment.

"Remember that case I was telling you about the other night? The one Singleton hooked me up with. There's a fourteen-year-old boy who was placed in a residential center for kids with serious emotional problems. His parents had a hard time getting help for him and they had to give custody of him to the state before DSS would pay for his treatment. It's a real mess. If that wasn't bad enough, he's been accused of killing another kid and his parents have asked me to find out what happened. I have to go to western Massachusetts for a few days, but I should be back after the weekend."

To my surprise Ollie's eyes lit up. "Are you going near Northampton? I've wanted to go back to Smith to see some of my professors. Would you mind if I tagged along? It would give us time to talk and I'd love to show you some of my old hangouts."

This was not like Ollie. Usually I was the one who pushed for us to travel. She was content to stay in central New York. And when it came to doing anything related to my investigative work, I practically had to beg her to accompany me. "Are you sure you want to come with me?"

"Positive. Traffic is slow at the museum and I have a few vacation days coming to me. I think it would be good for us to get away from here for awhile."

Ollie's enthusiasm for coming with me to Massachusetts caught me off guard. Even after her explanation I was still somewhat puzzled. But spending a few days with her might help us sort through our problems. We might even have some fun. Besides, I'd probably spend a lot of time worrying about why she was angry at me if she didn't come.

We agreed that I would pick her up at eight-thirty the next morning. By that time the twenty-minute Syracuse rush hour would be over. With any luck we would get to Northampton in time for lunch.

CHAPTER SIX

The staff here is mean. They don't ask me what I want to do. They always tell me be quiet. It's not fun here. At least they were nice to me sometimes at the other place. I want to go home.

There is a short stretch of the New York Thruway, just east of Utica, where it is always snowing. The dark gray nimbostratus clouds, pushed along by the Canadian jet stream, soak up moisture as they cross Lake Ontario. Once clear of the lake these clouds, stimulated by the colder air, relieve their swollen bladders, dumping heavy wet snowflakes on the flat, monotonous landscape through which the highway passes.

I have encountered snowdrifts on this strip of road in April and ice patches in early October. Once, flying to Boston, I looked down and saw a dense band of snow falling on the same section of the thruway. The sun shone brightly on both sides of the snow.

This trip was no exception. Huge white snowflakes fell from the sky. Fortunately, the air temperature was warm enough to keep the flakes from posing a threat. The swirling snow and the whirring sound of the windshield wipers seemed to have a cathartic effect on Ollie. As soon as we entered the squall she began to talk about our relationship.

At first she went over the same ground we had covered yesterday, telling me how puzzled she was by her feelings of resentment toward me. My last attempt to use my psychological skills to help Ollie express herself had been such a dismal failure that I suppressed my urge to try another therapeutic intervention. Instead I focused on keeping the car on the road and listened attentively as Ollie struggled to make sense of her feelings. After a few minutes she stopped talking and sat silently, looking straight ahead. When I glanced over I noticed tears welling up in her eyes. Not wanting to embarrass her I looked away, but not soon enough. She turned toward me and sighed. "I'm sorry," she said softly. "I guess I've been kidding myself. I knew I was angry at you and I convinced myself I didn't know why. I guess I didn't want to face it."

Now I was really confused . . . and becoming more nervous by the second.

"I'm sorry, Marty," she said, dabbing at her eyes with a tissue. "I'm not ready for a serious relationship. You seem to be, but I'm not. As much as you say that you're willing to just enjoy my company and not worry about the future, it doesn't come across that way. You're just not that kind of person."

"But..."

"No, let me finish. You told me you've spent most of your life trying to stay away from long-term commitments, but when you met me all of that changed. I have no reason to doubt you. In fact, I believe that you are ready to settle down. I also know that once you make up your mind to do something you won't quit until you've done it. In some ways I admire that quality in you. But it can also be annoying, especially when you act as if you've changed your course when you really haven't."

This time I couldn't keep quiet. "Wait a minute. How can you know what I want? Are you some kind of mind reader? I meant it when I said I would back off. I've been working real hard to take things one day at a time. This isn't fair, Ollie."

"Maybe not. But that doesn't change how I feel. Up until today I wasn't even sure what I felt. But just a minute ago, as I was telling you how confused I was, it suddenly made sense to me. This image, or more accurately daydream, flashed into my head. You were standing at my door with a nice bouquet of flowers. Instead of handing them to me you were shoving them in my face and I couldn't breathe. I was really mad at you for sticking the flowers in my face, but I didn't do anything about it. I didn't tell you to take them away, I didn't push you. I just stood there being angry. Finally, I stepped back a few feet. I was able to breathe again and immediately stopped feeling angry."

"But I haven't given you flowers in months," I said, knowing as I spoke that my literal interpretation was a pathetic attempt to distract

Ollie from her inevitable conclusion.

Mercifully she chose not to respond to my comment. "What I realized," she continued, "is that I've been acting like a coward. Rather than taking responsibility for my own discomfort—or even more to the point, my passivity in dealing with this situation I've been blaming you. And for what? For caring for me and wanting to have a normal long-term relationship. The more I avoid dealing with this, the angrier I become with you."

I couldn't get rid of the image of me sticking flowers in Ollie's face, but I was relieved to hear her say she didn't blame me. Not completely relieved, however. "If you're not ready for a serious relationship," I said, "what do you want?"

Ollie continued to stare straight ahead. She took a tissue from her purse and blew her nose. Crumpling the tissue in her hand, she turned to me and said softly, "I don't know. I just don't know."

The despair in her voice triggered a sudden sense of sadness in me. As I struggled to hold back my tears I realized how foolish I had been. How could I think that I could convince Ollie to commit to a long term-relationship with me? If I had been in her place I would have turned and run at the first sign of being backed into a corner. I should have known better. Ollie was nothing if not independent. If she wanted some space, she should have it, no questions asked, no explanation needed.

Only one question remained. If I was so analytic, so rational, how come tears were streaming down my cheeks?

"You want to pull off the road, Marty?" Ollie asked.

"Nah. I'll be okay," I lied.

Ollie turned in her seat and patted my shoulder. Ordinarily I would have welcomed her expression of concern, probably even encouraged her to comfort me. But I was too upset to appreciate her gesture. She had thrown me a curveball and I had been too stunned to duck. I wasn't going to give her the satisfaction of knowing how much she had hurt me and how much I wanted to be with her.

If I had thought about it I would have realized how stupid my reaction was. But at that moment I was too absorbed in self-pity to care about the quality of my logic. I pivoted away from Ollie, pretending to notice something at the side of the road. She removed her hand from my shoulder and returned it to her lap.

For the next hour we drove in silence. Predictably the snow flurries stopped as we passed the Utica exit. In a few miles the clouds gave way to blue sky and bright sunshine.

Under other circumstances it would have been a nice day.

As we approached Schenectady I asked Ollie if she wanted to stop at the rest area. She said she was okay and thanked me for asking. The next time we spoke was on Route 91, in Massachusetts, when I asked her which of the Northampton exits we should take. The only thing that made the trip marginally tolerable was Harry Chapin's Gold Medal Collection. It was the only music we both liked and as much as I was tempted to play something she didn't like, the thought of generating even a tiny amount of additional conflict was enough to make me select Harry's tapes.

We rolled down the exit ramp and turned left on Route 5. My first impression of Northampton was not very positive. Ollie had always raved about what a fantastic town it was. Great restaurants, wonderful bookstores, always something to do. What I saw were some rundown houses, a couple of seedy stores, and a gas station. As we approached a large intersection, Ollie suggested I find a parking spot. I pulled onto a side street and found a spot in a parking lot at the rear of a row of old brick buildings. Another abandoned manufacturing town, I thought. Was it shoes or industrial machinery or baby food? They had all gone south—literally. The unions' hard won battle for decent wages had proved to be a hollow victory as companies were lured to the sunny South by low wages, tax breaks and other economic incentives. Now of course, many of these same businesses were relocating once again to Asia and Latin America as states scrambled frantically to attract companies drawn to the cheap labor of third-world countries.

Unfortunately the high-tech enterprises that were revitalizing some sections of the Northeast were not locating where the factories had been. Many of the old manufacturing towns had never recovered.

We locked the car and set out to find a restaurant. I noticed that Ollie had more spring in her step. I was not ready to share her excitement at returning to her alma mater. I was still smarting from the bomb she had dropped on me a few hours ago. I was getting ready to make a snide comment about the dilapidated condition of her wonderful college town when we turned the corner onto the main street and my impression of Northampton changed abruptly.

The sidewalk was packed with people, mostly young men and women engaged in animated conversation. The old brick buildings, which appeared so drab and ugly from the rear, looked quite different in front. Small shops of every variety lined both sides of the street. Books, clothing, music, jewelry, athletic gear. And food. There were more ethnic restaurants crammed into those rows of buildings than one might find in a considerably larger city.

I turned to tell Ollie that I was impressed, but she was not there. I spotted her halfway up the block, moving at a brisk pace. By the time I caught up with her she had turned the corner and was standing in front of a pizza place.

"It's gone," she said, frowning.

"What's gone?" I said, trying to catch my breath.

"Spoleto."

"What's a Spoleto?" I asked.

"An Italian restaurant. It had great food and the servings were huge. I used to save my money until I had enough to treat myself to dinner. It wasn't expensive, but I couldn't afford to eat there more than two or three times a semester. I would stuff myself until I felt I wouldn't be able to eat for a week. Unfortunately I was always hungry the next day."

"Did other people share your good opinion of Spoleto?"

"Oh yes. It was always packed. On Saturday night you might wait an hour for a table."

"That's odd," I said. "You would think that a good restaurant could survive in a college town like this, even though things have changed a lot in the twenty years since you graduated."

Ollie poked me on the arm as she said, "We're not all senior citizens."

My arm hurt where she hit me, but I was glad that we had exchanged quips. It eased the tension between us, if only for the moment.

"Any other good places to eat?" I asked. "Traveling always makes me hungry."

Ollie grinned. "Welcome to paradise. There probably isn't a bad place to eat in Northampton, at least there wasn't when I was at Smith *seven* years ago. What are you in the mood for?"

"Actually all of that talk about Italian food has given me a craving for pizza."

"I don't know about this place, but there's a good place around the corner."

"Let's do it."

Ollie guided us to Pinocchio's, a tiny pizzeria in the middle of the main strip, where I had a delicious slice of artichoke pizza and a Snapple. After we had eaten we split up. Ollie wanted to wander around the campus while I met with the prosecutor and tried to contact the lawyer Hannigan had recommended. We agreed to meet later in the afternoon at the ice cream shop across the street. It was apparent to me that whatever else happened on our trip to western Massachusetts, we would eat well.

Roger Darrow, the assistant district attorney handling Tommy's case, was a well dressed, stocky man in his early to mid-thirties. To compensate for his thinning hair he had let the few remaining strands grow long and combed them across the top of his head. In spite of his concern with physical appearance Darrow did not come across as a pretentious person.

"Welcome to the Pioneer Valley, Mr. Fenton," he said, greeting me with a firm handshake. "And in case you're wondering, I'm not related to Clarence."

It took me a second to figure out what he was saying. I tried to think of a smart retort but drew a blank. Probably not worth pursuing anyway, especially since I needed his cooperation.

"Your client's in a rough spot," Darrow said, shaking his head. "I can't imagine having to give my kid up to the state in order to get help. It must be hell for them, especially with the kid being in big trouble."

"You've got that right," I said, trying to fit in with Darrow's colloquial style. "They're feeling pretty damn helpless." I didn't know why I was talking that way. It must have been something I picked up in one of my psych books: *Identifying with the other member of the communication dyad facilitates open dialogue.* Or something like that.

"So what can I do for you," Darrow said, gesturing me toward a group of armchairs clustered around a coffee table in the far corner of his office. After settling himself in a chair across from me, he offered me a mint from the glass dish on the coffee table. "You must have gone through some hoops to get the judge to allow you to represent the parents. That privilege is usually reserved for barristers like me."

"It took a little effort," I said, smiling. "Let's just say I had some help from another member of your esteemed profession." More of that mimic talk. I really had to watch myself.

"What exactly does the judge's order say?"

I reached into my pocket and handed him the order. He studied it for a moment, then returned it to me. "Looks like the genuine article," Darrow said. "I'll get you the police report. While you're reading the report I'll call over to the detention home and let them know you're coming to visit the Hammond boy. I need to warn you though, I don't think you'll get much help from him."

"Why's that?"

"He isn't a real talkative chap. He seems more interested in studying the tops of his shoes than talking to other people." Darrow rose from his chair and walked to the door.

"Thanks for the warning," I said, impressed by the prosecutor's congeniality. I had anticipated a less friendly reception.

At the door, Darrow turned to me and said, "By the way, I hope you enjoy some of Northampton's fine cuisine while you're here. It's about the only satisfaction you're likely to have. We've got the kid dead to rights. When you read the police report you'll see what I mean. Enjoy your stay." Darrow gave me a broad smile and left the room before I had a chance to respond.

Maybe the assistant district attorney wasn't as congenial as he first appeared.

After a few moments a pencil-thin gray-haired woman appeared. She escorted me to a small cubicle at the end of the corridor. Before relinquishing the brown folder she clutched to her bosom, she cautioned me not to write on, copy, remove or tamper with in any way the contents of the folder. She did not explicitly tell me I would be caned, castrated or stood in front of a firing squad if I so much as smudged any of the pages, but her tone left no doubt in my mind. I was being entrusted with an official document and she would be checking to make sure I handled the file with the respect it was due.

It was a thin file containing Tommy's booking sheet and a two page report submitted by the officer who had responded to the call from the treatment center. In spite of its brevity, the report contained ample information to support Darrow's confidence about the case against Tommy.

When the officer arrived at the center he was brought directly to the room where the dead boy had been found. Upon entering the room he immediately noticed the body of a small boy lying face down on the floor next to a bed. The boy's arms were spread out to the side and his right leg was crossed over his left leg. The officer noted his first impression of the body, stating that he looked like someone who had been nailed backward to a crucifix. There was a dark stain on the floor next to the boy's body, which the officer later confirmed to be blood.

Sitting on the bed on the other side of the room was another small, disheveled boy who appeared to be staring at the floor. The boy on the bed was holding a blood-stained hunting knife.

The only other person in the room was a supervisor who was trying to remain calm as he pleaded with the boy to put down the knife.

The boy lying in the pool of blood was Kevin Landry. He was thirteen years old and lived in the room in which he was found. The boy holding the knife was Tommy Hammond, who lived next door.

The remainder of the report documented the supervisor's story of how he found Kevin and Tommy, and the police officer's modest account of how he successfully persuaded Tommy to drop the hunting knife into an evidence bag.

Remembering the pencil woman's admonition about Tommy's file I gently placed the report back into the folder, being careful not to crease the pages. Fearing there might be a rule about removing the file from the document examination room, I stuck my head outside the cubicle, hoping to find someone who would relieve me of my burden. No such luck. There was no one in the hallway.

I tiptoed out of the cubicle and had almost reached the other end of the corridor when I heard someone behind me clear their throat. The sound startled me and I spun around. Standing in front of the cubicle I had just occupied was the Keeper of the File, arms folded in front of her, glaring at me as if I had just abducted her firstborn. I hadn't heard a door open and I was certain no one had been in the corridor.

"I'll take that if you're through," she said icily.

I thrust the file into her hands, mumbled my appreciation for her help and left before she had a chance to examine the file. I knew it was not damaged but I still felt guilty.

Although they bore no resemblance to each other I wondered whether the pencil woman was related to my mother.

The police report had been about as uplifting as my conversation with Ollie on the trip from Syracuse. I was hoping for a more muddled scenario. But finding Tommy with a knife in his hand sitting across from the dead boy did not leave room for a lot of alternative explanations.

I found a pay phone and tried the lawyer again. The woman who answered had a husky voice with a distinct Boston accent. She identified herself as Faith Pasternak and told me she could see me if I came to her office right away. Her office was in a three-story building behind the courthouse. It was a red brick building that housed a restaurant and an upscale women's clothing store on the ground floor. The directory in the narrow entryway listed four tenants: a social worker and nutritionist on the second floor, and Ms. Pasternak, Esq., and an accountant on the top floor. One-stop shopping. You could get your mind and body fixed up, straighten out your finances and if you had any money left, retain an attorney to help you with your legal problems.

I took the elevator to the third floor and knocked on the frosted glass door whose slightly crooked gold letters announced that this was the office of Faith Pasternak, Attorney-At-Law. I knocked twice and when no one answered I opened the door.

The reception room was small and sparsely furnished: a walnut desk with a telephone and electric typewriter, three metal and vinyl arm chairs, and a dark wooden coffee table that almost matched the desk. A far cry from Jerome Hannigan's elegant front office.

"Hello," I said, moving toward the only one of the three doors that was open.

"In here, Mr. Fenton." It was the voice of the woman on the telephone and it came from the room I was walking toward. I stuck my head into the doorway, but did not see anyone. The room was larger than I expected considering the cramped hallway and tiny reception room. The office opened to the left. The far wall was lined with waist-high bookshelves filled with leather-bound law books. Straight ahead was a round table with three chairs. Behind this was a long L-shaped work space attached to the wall. The work space was cluttered with papers and books. On the right were a telephone, computer, and printer. Above the computer were several framed diplomas and on the wall facing the door was a narrow window covered by a maroon curtain. The only light in the room was a fluorescent fixture on the wall directly above the work space.

Hearing a whirring sound to my left I turned to see a small woman in an electric wheelchair emerge from a narrow alcove beyond the bookshelves. Her thin, pale face was framed by a helmet of silver hair cut in a straight line just below her jaw line. It was difficult to tell how old she was. Her strong voice certainly belied her frail appearance.

"It's a pleasure to meet you, Mr. Fenton," she said as she wheeled toward me. She stopped her chair in front of me and held out her hand. I bent down and took her tiny hand and was surprised by how warm it was. "I'm Faith Pasternak, though Rudy Flores, my accountant next door, tells me I should change my name to Charity based on my billing practices. Welcome to my humble suite. A little unorthodox but functional. Can I get you something to drink?"

"Oh, I don't want to put you to any trouble."

She cocked her head and looked at me, but didn't say anything. I immediately felt like a jerk. "Actually I am a little thirsty," I said sheepishly. "What do you have?"

"Almost anything a normal person might drink. Coffee, tea, soft drinks, water from the underground springs at Lourdes."

"Look, I'm sorry. You took me by surprise. I'm usually not such a schmuck."

"So?"

I couldn't think of anything more to say. I felt as if I would just get myself in deeper. "What do you want me to say?"

"You could start by telling me what you want to drink." We both laughed and I was grateful to her for breaking the tension.

While Faith returned to the alcove to get coffee for both of us. I looked at the certificates on the wall. B.A. with high honors from Mount Holyoke. Member of Phi Beta Kappa. Ph.D. in political science from Yale.

Doctor of Jurisprudence from Harvard Law School.

"My mother wanted me to hang up my Girl Scout badges but I had to draw the line somewhere," Faith said, taking two cups from the tray on her wheelchair and placing them on the round table. "How's Jerry? I haven't seen him in years."

I had to think for a moment, but finally figured out she meant Jerome Hannigan. "I guess he's okay. I don't really know him well. He was reluctant to take on this case. In fact, he was pretty peeved at me for stretching the truth when I called for an appointment. I told him I had a problem, which is partly true, because my client's problem is also my problem. When I told him I had made an appointment with him because of the Hammonds' problem he was not happy. He really laid me out."

Faith chuckled. "I'm surprised he didn't take your head off. Jerry has a short fuse when he feels someone's taking advantage of him. When we were at Harvard—he and I were in the same class in law school—he had a well-deserved reputation as someone you didn't mess with. One time a classmate borrowed Jerry's class notes for the Constitutional Law exam and conveniently forgot to bring them back to class the day before the test. Jerry was number two in the class and this guy was number three, close on his heels. The person ranked second gets to be associate editor of the law review."

"What happened?"

"Jerry had a long talk with this guy after class. He didn't raise his voice or make any threatening gestures, but when the other student walked by those of us who were unobtrusively eavesdropping, he was as white as a ghost. Twenty minutes later he returned with the notes. Jerry became associate editor and I occasionally wondered whether our pale-faced classmate knew more about Constitutional law than he wrote on that exam."

"Sounds like Mr. Hannigan is one tough guy," I said, grateful that I had gotten off so easily.

"Tough but fair. Jerry would go out of his way to help you as long as you were straight with him. He's always had a soft spot for the underdog. That's what makes him such a good attorney."

"Yeah, but what about all of those heavy hitters he represents? The corporate crooks, the members of the family?"

Faith looked down at her coffee. After a few seconds she looked at me and sighed. "I don't know. I wish I had a good answer to give you but I don't." She took a sip of coffee, then picked up a pen and legal pad. "Now why don't you tell me about Tommy Hammond?"

I wanted to know more about Jerome Hannigan. I wanted to find out how this frail looking, husky voiced woman with the impressive credentials on the wall had come to practice law in a dark, bare-bones office in Northampton, Massachusetts. I wanted to ask her who had been number one in their law school class. But I sensed the moment had passed and I knew that Tommy Hammond desperately needed our help.

Faith asked me to move my chair over to the work space. She rolled her chair up to the computer and motioned me to sit beside her. As I recounted what I knew about Tommy Hammond, beginning with my initial discussion with Professor Barker and ending with my review of his police file less than an hour earlier, Faith clicked away nonstop on the keyboard. When I finished my story she asked me if there was anything else I could recall. I told her there wasn't, she shook her head then tapped the *save* key and rolled her chair back from the computer.

"It doesn't look good for young Mr. Hammond," she said, turning her chair to face me.

"Not at all," I agreed. "The police report puts him at the scene of the crime with the body at his feet and the bloody weapon in his hand. Any chance the report is fabricated?"

"I don't know much about the staff at Possum Ridge," she replied. "It has a decent reputation. I'm pretty confident the police handled the investigation by the book. Law enforcement in the Valley is top notch. Very professional. With the concentration of young people from the five colleges in this area and the large number of tourists who are drawn to our scenic beauty and good food, we are a high-risk environment. The colleges have their own police officers, but once the students venture off campus they become easy targets. The same applies to tourists. Crime statistics have been on the rise here as they are just about everywhere. Several years ago the Chamber of Commerce became concerned that the crime problem would scare away vacationers. They convinced local officials to upgrade police services. It wasn't so much the crime itself. Communities can tolerate a fair amount of criminal activity. It was the potential loss of rои cпuе that spurred them to action. Money is a powerful motivator."

"I can understand the tourist business," I said, "but what did the college students have to do with it? My experience has been that the town doesn't care much about the gown and vice versa. Besides, kids rarely choose their colleges based on how safe the surrounding community is. If they did, schools like Columbia, Penn, and Yale would have been out of business a long time ago."

"You're right," Faith responded. "Up to a point. The colleges and the community have a symbiotic relationship. There's no love lost between them but they recognize that they need each other. The combined payrolls of the five schools far surpass any other employer in the area, not to mention the big bucks students spend with local merchants. Administrators at the colleges aren't naive enough to expect locals to welcome students with open arms, but they do expect them to keep the kids safe. And when some of the young people have too much to drink and become a little rowdy, college officials count on the local police to handle the situation discreetly."

"What about Darrow?" I asked. "What kind of guy is he?"

"His Mr. Nice Guy routine grates on my nerves but otherwise he's competent and ethical, at least for a prosecutor."

"Looks like we've got our work cut out for us," I said gloomily.

"You're a master of understatement," Faith said as she propelled her chair toward the alcove. "Give me a minute and we'll be ready to go."

"Where are we going?" I asked, hoping at least one of us knew what she was doing.

"To see our client, of course," Faith replied as she disappeared into the alcove.

CHAPTER SEVEN

One thing I like here is they leave the light on at night. At the other place they make us turn all the lights out when we go to bed. One night I get real upset. I tell them I'm scared but they don't listen. The big man comes to see me. After that they let me keep a light on.

Faith's van was a tribute to modern technology. With a zap of her remote control the side door slid open and a chairlift glided out and down to the ground. Faith wheeled herself onto the lift and locked the wheels. She zapped again and the lift rose up and slid into the van. Once inside, she pushed another button and the driver's seat swiveled to the side, allowing her to transfer from her wheelchair to the seat.

In addition to a special set of hand controls for accelerating and braking, the driver's compartment had a series of buttons and levers whose functions I could only guess. There was a speaker phone built into the dashboard and a panel of dials that rivaled the cockpit of a Boeing 737. There was even a small compartment that looked as if it were made to hold a small notebook computer.

Sitting in the passenger's seat, watching Faith getting ready to drive the van, I suddenly felt guilty for all of the times I had expressed frustration for the petty inconveniences of driving. How could I compare my annoyance at having to add a quart of oil or clean the windshield with the preparation required just to turn on the ignition of this vehicle? I made a mental note to remember this the next time an "out of order" sign forced me to move to another gas pump.

As we were pulling out of the parking space she turned to me. "The detention center is about twenty-five miles from here. I prefer to take the side roads rather than the interstate. I hope you don't mind."

I was curious about why she didn't want to take the highway but decided not to ask. Instead I added her preference for the scenic route to the growing list of questions I had about Faith Pasternak.

The regional detention center was a long, one-story, cinder block building. The parking lot was in the rear. On one side of the building was a small patch of grass equipped with volleyball net and a pair of basketball goal posts. It could have passed for a recreation center if not for the high barbed wire fence that encircled the property.

Once inside my impression quickly changed. The surly guard at the security check point seemed put out by Faith's wheelchair. He insisted that she pass through the metal detector gate. Not only did the chair become stuck, the metal fixtures activated the warning signal.

Faith patiently tolerated the guard's belligerent manner until he announced that he would have to remove her from the chair to check for weapons. Then she told him he was welcome to do so, but should be prepared to answer charges that he had violated a number of federal statutes and would need to tend to the scratches she would place on his face if he tried. The guard decided to call his supervisor.

After a quick assessment of the situation the supervisor, a tall wiry man with slicked back hair, apologized to Faith for any inconvenience she had experienced and told us he would take us to see Tommy. Bypassing the security gate we walked through a small waiting room into a dimly lit intersection of three corridors. The center hallway appeared to be lined with offices; to the left and right large metal doors limited access to the other corridors. The supervisor led us to the door on the right.

"The kids are placed by age and gender," the supervisor explained, reaching into his pocket. "Boys sixteen and over are housed on the other unit. The younger boys and the females—we usually don't get too many of them—stay on this unit. Once in awhile we have a situation involving a male and female but never anything too serious. Funny thing is, it's always the females who provoke the situation."

Using an oversized skeleton key, the kind I've seen in the movies about Alcatraz, he opened the door and led us into a large room. He quickly closed the door and turned the key. The sound of the lock snapping shut startled me and I instinctively stepped toward the door. The supervisor glanced at me but didn't say anything. I suspected it was not the first time he had seen that reaction.

"This is the day room," the supervisor said pointing to the large, sparsely furnished room we were standing in. "The kids are pretty much free to do what they want—as long as it's legal," he chuckled.

Judging from the room's facilities, the residents were not at risk of being overwhelmed by the options available to them. In addition to several heavy wooden sofas—bolted to the floor—there were two round tables with attached benches. Seated at one of the tables was a group of young adolescent boys engrossed in a game of cards. The other table was occupied by a trio of teenage girls working on their hair and nails. Several boys sat on the sofas reading comic books and one little boy, who couldn't have been more than eight, sat on the floor playing with a piece of paper folded into the shape of an airplane. Presumably supervising the children were a large black woman and a short white man who stood at opposite sides of the room, arms folded in front, periodically scanning the room.

The supervisor waved to the staff, who nodded but did not interrupt their surveillance. Several of the youngsters took an interest in us, especially Faith.

"You here to see me?" asked a thin black girl.

"No, Yolanda," the supervisor replied. "I told you this morning your P.O. isn't coming until tomorrow."

"Well I thought they might be some other folks who wanted to talk wif me."

The little boy playing with the paper plane pointed to Faith and asked, "What's wrong with her?"

The supervisor pointed his finger at the boy. "Not your business, Ricky. You've got enough trouble of your own to worry about." Turning to us he said, "The kids have teachers that come in a couple hours a day. State law. They also have forty-five minutes a day recreation in the courtyard."

"How long do the children stay here?" I asked.

The supervisor shrugged. "It all depends. Some of them for a couple of days. Others might be here a few months 'til their disposition is settled. One kid was with us almost ten months because his lawyer screwed up."

I looked at Faith, but she seemed oblivious to what the supervisor was saying. Her gaze was fixed on a short boy with curly red hair who was looking at a comic book. I couldn't tell whether she recognized the boy or was simply trying to fathom something about him. Whatever the intent, her gaze was intense.

Abruptly Faith broke her concentration and turned to our host. "Which one is Tommy Hammond?"

"Oh, he's not here," the supervisor said. "Because of his situation we have him on SP."

"SP?" I asked. I had figured out that P.O. stood for probation officer, but I was stumped by SP.

The supervisor puffed up his skinny chest and proceeded to educate us about detention center terminology. "It stands for special precautions but it's really a polite way to let staff know they better protect the administration's butt. A kid like Tommy, there's no tellin' what he might do. Might find something sharp to cut himself with. Might try to hang himself. Kid like Tommy does himself in, you're lookin' at front page headlines and special investigations for a month of Sundays."

I was interested in hearing more about the empathic procedures of the detention center but I could see by the way Faith was moving in her chair that she was anxious to see Tommy. "Where is Tommy?" I asked.

"Follow me," the supervisor said leading us to the rear of the day room where there was a row of doors on each side. Behind each door was a bedroom decorated in the same charming mode as the day room. A few of the rooms contained a single bed and built-in dresser; most were furnished for double occupancy. The bedroom doors were also made of metal and each had a small square window at about eye level. My guess was that the windows were not made of ordinary glass.

At the end of one hallway another support staff member stood in front of a closed door. As we approached, the supervisor called to the man, "Barry, these folks are here to see Tommy Hammond. The lady is his lawyer and I'm not sure who this guy is, but he's got a judge's order says he can visit the boy. Give them some privacy but don't take your eyes off the kid."

"You got it," Barry said, saluting the supervisor. As he opened the door the supervisor wished us good luck and told us he would be in his office if we needed him. Before leaving he pulled Barry aside and whispered in

69

his ear.

This room was even more barren than the others. While it might not technically qualify as a padded cell, thick floor-to-ceiling mats lined the walls. The only outside light came from a narrow horizontal window in the upper corner of the room. The only furniture was a covered mattress lying on the floor next to the back wall. Sitting cross-legged on the mattress, head hanging down, was a frail-looking child who I assumed to be Tommy Hammond. He certainly didn't look anything like the little boy with the crooked smile in Ruth Hammond's photo album.

"Visitors, Tommy," Barry said as we entered. "He isn't much for talking," he whispered. The boy on the mattress didn't acknowledge our presence. Strands of long, oily black hair hung over his face. From where I stood I couldn't tell whether his eyes were open or closed. His thin arms protruded from a plain white T-shirt and he wore a pair of baggy jeans. His feet, which seemed small even for a person of his stature, were bare.

We waited a moment, hoping he would at least look at us. When he didn't, Faith inched forward and addressed him.

"I'm Faith Pasternak and I'm an attorney. Your parents have hired me to represent you. This is Marty Fenton. He's a private investigator and he's also here to help you." Faith paused, but the boy did not respond. "Your parents are quite concerned about you," she continued. "They will be coming to visit you this weekend."

The boy lifted his head slowly. His eyes, dark orbs in hollow sockets, were both intense and flat at once. Filled with anger, even rage, they seemed to repel any attempt to make contact. The gate separating the outside of his body from the inside was shut tight. He wasn't going to let anyone in and anything that mattered to him was unlikely to see the light of day.

As Professor Ormsby, my abnormal psychology teacher, used to say, Tommy Hammond would definitely fail the peeper test.

Tommy glanced at Faith, then turned toward the wall.

"Don't care," he mumbled.

Faith leaned forward in her chair. "That's hard for me to believe," she said softly. "Here you are stuck in a padded room facing charges that you killed another boy and you don't care if your parents come to see you. Sorry, Tommy, I'm not buying that."

"Not *me*," Tommy said.

"This is no time to go macho on us, young man," Faith said, the tone kinder than her words. "You're in serious trouble and you need all the help you can get."

Suddenly Tommy lurched toward Faith and screamed, "Not me. Not me, don't care. Them." Barry quickly moved in to restrain Tommy, but Faith, her face only inches from the troubled boy's face, raised her hand signaling Barry to remain where he was.

"Who is 'them'?" she asked quietly.

Hovering over the diminutive attorney, Tommy did not respond. His eyes were glazed and a thin string of saliva dangled from the corner of his mouth. Barry leaned forward, ready to spring into action. I stood behind Barry hoping that Tommy would sit back on his mattress.

After a long moment of silence Faith reached up and cupped the boy's face in her small hands. Barry and I tensed, waiting for Tommy to react. But he didn't.

"I'm sorry," Faith said softly. "I misunderstood you. I can see why you might think your parents don't care about you. Anyone would feel like that if they were in your situation. But your mom and dad didn't want to put you here. They felt like they didn't have a choice. They couldn't take care of you at home and they want you to get better. This was their only option."

Tommy looked at Faith for a second then sat down on his mattress and resumed looking at the wall.

"Whether you believe it or not, Mr. Fenton and I are here to help you," Faith said. "We're going to need to know what happened at Possum Ridge; what happened to Kevin, why you had a knife in your hand and whether anyone else was involved. If you want to tell us anything now I can ask Barry to step outside. If you're not ready to talk now that's okay, also. We'll come back later. What do you say, Tommy?"

Tommy continued to stare at the wall.

After a moment we said goodbye to Tommy and told him we'd be back the next day. In the hallway Barry said to Faith, "You're one brave lady. I know a lot of bigger people, myself included, who wouldn't have had the guts to lay their hands on Tommy the way you did."

Ignoring his comment Faith said, "I want to see the supervisor. Would you please take us to him now?"

Barry looked over at me and raised his eyebrows. "I didn't mean to insult you," he said to Faith. "I just think that you were pretty gutsy."

"Don't worry," Faith responded. "My request to see the supervisor has nothing to do with you."

As we entered his office the supervisor stood. "I hope your visit was . . ."

"If you want to know if I was satisfied with my visit the answer is no," Faith said. "Tommy Hammond is not receiving appropriate care. You have him locked in a padded cell. With the exception of staff occasionally peeking through the window in the door, he is not getting personal attention and from what I can see he has not received medical care since he was admitted to your facility."

The supervisor's face turned pink. "Listen, that boy was put in here because he stabbed another boy with a knife. Not just stabbed him. He killed that boy. You can see for yourself that he's not all there. No tellin' what he might do. Our job is to keep everyone in our custody safe—the kids and the staff—and that's exactly what we're doing."

By now I knew that Faith was not likely to respond well to the supervisor's remarks. She leaned forward, as if she was going to step out of her wheelchair. "I've got no problem with your goals; it's how you're trying to achieve them that concerns me. I suggest, Mr. . . I'm sorry, I didn't get your name."

The supervisor's face was now crimson. "Helfinger. Donald B. Helfinger. I've worked in this facility for eighteen years, been supervisor for the last eleven. You can check the evaluation sheets—mine and the facility's. Clean as a baby's bottom."

Now I don't claim to be an expert in child rearing. My experience is limited to watching my sister's eighteen-month-old while she took her older child to the doctor. But even I cringed at Helfinger's metaphor.

"Look, Mr. Helfinger," Faith said, sitting back in her chair. "I'm not here to give you a hard time. I'm sure you're a conscientious administrator, trying to do the best job you can. I just want you to understand the legal ramifications of what's going on here."

The telephone on Helfinger's desk rang and he reached for it quickly, grateful for the distraction. From Helfinger's tone, the person on the other end of the line must have had some stature. He didn't address the individual by name, but was exceedingly deferential, using the word "sir" at least once in every sentence. The caller was obviously talking about one of the detention center's residents. Helfinger's responses were deliberately vague, limiting himself to "yes" or "no" answers whenever possible, not mentioning the resident's name. A more generous observer would have given him credit for protecting his charges' right to privacy. At that moment I was not inclined toward generosity. Faith looked at me with raised eyebrows. We were both thinking the same thing.

When Helfinger replaced the receiver I asked, "Have there been many calls about Tommy?"

"We get calls about all the kids," he replied.

"What kind of people call?" I asked, hoping a less direct approach would yield better results.

"All kinds," Helfinger said, letting me know that my strength did not lay in conducting probing interviews.

Mercifully, Faith took me off the hook. "As I was saying before we were interrupted, there are several legalities that shouldn't be overlooked. First, we need to remember that Tommy was placed in your custody because he is *alleged* to have stabbed Kevin. The issue of whether he actually killed this boy will be resolved in a court of law. Until that time he is presumed to be innocent."

The color was returning to Helfinger's cheeks. "I didn't mean to . . ."

"I'm sure your intentions are benevolent," Faith said. "I just want to make sure we're all clear about the legal context. Which brings me to my second point."

Helfinger rearranged the papers on his desk. I made a mental note to ask Faith for some pointers on effective communication.

"It doesn't take a board certified psychiatrist to see that Tommy is a seriously disturbed youngster who needs to be under the care of a mental health professional. If I'm not mistaken, section sixty-eight of chapter one-hundred-nineteen of the General Laws of the Commonwealth gives the court authority to detain a child charged with a serious crime in your facility. If this child shows evidence of having an emotional disorder he or she has a right to be evaluated immediately by a qualified psychiatrist or psychologist to determine the youth's mental status and the most appropriate course of treatment. Unless I'm mistaken, neither Barry nor any other member of your staff I have encountered possesses the appropriate credentials to conduct such an examination."

Helfinger glanced at Faith, then returned his attention to the papers on his desk. "Anything else, Ms. Pasternak?"

"No, other than to remind you of Tommy's right to legal counsel whenever he is to be questioned. But I'm sure I don't have to remind you of that."

"No, Ma'am."

"Good. Then we'll look forward to hearing the results of Tommy's psychiatric exam when we return, tomorrow."

Faith held out her hand. Helfinger leaned over his desk and cautiously shook it. He ignored my outstretched hand.

Barry escorted us from Helfinger's office to the security gate. I kept thinking he was going to say something, but he didn't. As soon as we were outside of hearing range I said to Faith, "You were great in there. I'm really impressed with your ability to communicate. The way you made contact with Tommy was remarkable. I don't think a mental health professional could have done better. And you certainly got your message across to Helfinger."

Faith chuckled nervously. "Thanks, but if you must know, I can't stand confrontational situations. If I had my choice I'd probably spend my time in a closet curled up in the fetal position. Maybe that's why I can identify with Tommy."

Her candid admission surprised me. "But . . . but isn't that what lawyers do, confront people?"

This time her laugh was more spontaneous. "I guess I'm a real shy attorney. It's pretty hard to cross-examine a witness with your thumb in your mouth."

"Why did you become a lawyer, if you don't like confrontation?"

"That's a long story. Better told over a pitcher of Margaritas. Suffice it to say for now that where I intended to go and where I eventually ended up were two distinctly different places."

Once again I was left with questions I was reluctant to ask.

On the ride back to town Faith gave me a brief cultural overview of the Pioneer Valley. Once a prosperous textile manufacturing center, it had struggled for survival after the factory owners exited to the South in search of inexpensive labor. Fortunately the Valley had been blessed with two more enduring assets. Its northern New England location attracted visitors year around: winter sports, the music and theater of the Berkshires in the summer, and the spectacular fall foliage brought a steady stream of visitors and their dollars to the area. The Valley's other asset was its institutions of higher education. Known as the five colleges, Amherst, Hampshire, Mount Holyoke, Smith, and the University of Massachusetts at Amherst brought jobs and consumers to the Holyoke-Amherst-Northampton area, not to mention considerable cultural enrichment and prestige.

As with all dependent relationships, the local community was ambivalent toward its source of sustenance. Complaining about the tourists and students was a favorite local pastime as was reminiscing about the good old days when everyone knew each other and there was no traffic to contend with.

Still there were no serious attempts to discourage the tourists or shut down the colleges. The taciturn folks who considered themselves to be the legitimate citizens of the Valley had too much New England common sense to tamper with the economic lifeline of the community.

Faith was describing the unique relationship between the community and its two single-sex colleges, Smith and Mt. Holyoke, when I heard the sound of an engine roaring behind us. Before I could turn to see the source of the noise, there was a loud thud and our van began to swerve. I saw a dark blur pass us on the left and at the same time heard the screech of brakes. Our van spun around several times and, as I clutched the armrest with all of my strength, I was convinced I was going to die.

After what seemed an eternity, but actually must have been no more than a few seconds, the car stopped twirling and slid off the road into a ditch where it bumped against a large tree and came to a halt.

When I was certain the van was no longer moving, I looked over at Faith and was shocked to see her slumped over the wheel. Her face was ashen gray and she was not moving. With my heart racing I reached over to feel her pulse. Before my hand reached her neck I heard a low moaning sound. At first I thought the sound was coming from behind me, but when the moan escalated to an ear piercing howl I knew that Faith was still alive.

I sat frozen in my seat, not knowing how to respond. If she was hurt, what could I do? The last first aid course I took was in the summer after my junior year of high school when I worked as a lifeguard at the YMCA. I didn't see any blood, but I was afraid that she might have broken some bones or, worse yet, sustained internal injuries.

Just as my anxiety was reaching panic level her scream became coherent: "No, no. Get up. You need to help me. Speak to me, dammit. I need your help."

"It's okay, Faith," I said. "I'll help you".

At the sound of my voice she stopped screaming and opened her eyes. She swiveled toward the back seat then turned toward me. She looked puzzled, as if she didn't expect to see me sitting next to her. When she recognized who I was her eyes welled up with tears and she began to sob. Awkwardly I reached over and tried to comfort her. Not knowing whether she was hurt and having no previous experience holding a woman who was wheelchair bound, my embrace was more tentative than I would have liked. Faith didn't seem to notice, however. She buried her face in my chest and cried. Her small body heaved in sorrow until there was nothing more to release. When her breathing finally returned to normal she looked up at me and smiled. "You must think I'm one crazy lady."

"Not at all," I replied. "I'm just glad that you're okay, that we're okay. We could have been killed."

"I know. I guess I'm lucky. And this time I don't think it was an accident."

"This time?"

"Oh, I'm sorry. I guess I owe you an explanation."

"You know why we were run off the road?"

"No, that's not what I mean. I don't know why we were sideswiped unless someone is unhappy about us speaking to Tommy Hammond. What I mean is you deserve to know why I reacted the way I did."

"It sounded like a pretty natural response to being run off the road," I lied. I wasn't sure I wanted to know what had triggered her grief.

"I'm making you uncomfortable, aren't I?" she said.

Damn, was I that transparent? "Maybe a little. But if you'd like to tell me, I'll be glad to listen."

Faith shook her head. "You sound more like a psychologist than a private investigator."

"That's another story," I said sheepishly. "Maybe I can tell you about me later."

"Okay. But first let's see if we can get this car back on the road."

I got out of the car to inspect the damage. There was a dent in the right front fender and the plastic headlight cover was cracked, but otherwise the van seemed to be okay. I climbed back into the van and told Faith what I had found. "Not bad for a dwarf paraplegic who's never made it over the first mountain on my PlayStation," she joked. Her face was no longer gray and her emotional state was definitely better.

She turned the ignition key and after a few anxious seconds the engine turned over. With a little maneuvering Faith had us back on the road.

On the drive back to Northampton she told me about her first accident. After hearing her story I understood why she had reacted so strongly when we were pushed off the road. I also had an answer to my earlier question about why she chose to avoid the interstate highway.

She spoke softly as she recounted what happened. At times I had to strain to understand what she was saying, but I was reluctant to ask her to speak up. Eleven years ago she was returning from a Thanksgiving visit with her parents in New Hampshire. At the time, she lived in Manhattan with her husband Zach and their four-year-old son Danny. She was working for a small firm that specialized in environmental law. Zach had just been made a partner in one of New York's most prestigious firms. As they crossed into Massachusetts it began to snow heavily. Visibility was poor and they considered stopping, but Zach had to be in court early the next day, so they decided to push on. Zach had spent his adolescence in Southern California and had gone to college in Berkeley. During his three years in Cambridge he hadn't owned a car. Faith had grown up in Lynn, Massachusetts and was used to driving in the snow. Zach, who had been driving, pulled off the road and turned the wheel over to Faith.

At this point in her story Faith sighed. She hesitated before continuing.

"Just north of Northampton on Route 91 we ran into a snow squall. The car ahead of us skidded into our lane. With almost zero visibility I didn't have much time to react. I managed to avoid a head on collision, but clipped the rear end of the other vehicle. Our car spun out of control and left the road. It plunged down an embankment, flipped over, and smashed into a tree.

"When the rescue squad finally came they had to cut off the driver's door to reach us. The car had hit the tree on the passenger's side and Zach's skull had been crushed. He was dead upon arrival. Danny, who had been lying on the back seat, was thrown against the side of the car. He sustained a serious head injury and was unconscious when the rescue squad found him."

By now Faith was barely whispering.

"I was pinned between the driver's seat and the steering wheel and remained conscious the entire time. I was taken with Danny to the hospital in Northampton where the doctors discovered that I had fractured my arm and damaged my spinal cord. They told me I was paralyzed below the waist and was lucky to be alive. With my husband dead and my son in a coma, I did not agree with the doctors' assessment of my fortune.

"They waited a week to let me know I would never walk again and two weeks before telling me Danny was brain dead. My physical recovery was progressing as well as could be expected, but emotionally I was still shaky and was not prepared to accept this inevitable conclusion. During the next few weeks I pleaded with Danny's physicians to try other treatment approaches. Given my fragile condition the medical staff was reluctant to confront me. They listened to my pleas and patiently explained the limitations of modern medicine. Finally, after three weeks of trying to ignore their gentle rebuttals, I accepted the dreadful fact that Danny would never recover. That night I sat by his side holding his hand, talking to him through my tears. In the morning I said goodbye to Danny. Then I told the doctor to disconnect the life support system."

The pain of recounting this terrible experience showed on her face. I reached over and put my hand on her shoulder. She managed to curl her lip into faint smile.

"For reasons I didn't fully understand at the time, I decided to remain in Northampton for rehabilitation. My firm gave me an extended leave and for the next five months I immersed myself in the hospital's intensive rehab program. The spinal injury had left me without the use of my legs, but fortunately did not affect my upper body. The staff worked with me to strengthen my arms, chest, and shoulders. I learned again how to execute the mundane activities of daily living that we take for granted: getting out of bed, using the toilet, crossing the street. Although I would eventually have a battery-operated wheelchair, the staff wanted me to be able to use a manual chair. Perhaps the hardest lesson was learning to deal with the ignorance and prejudices of the ambulatory community, with all of the physical and psychological obstacles it erects to those of us with physical handicaps."

Her description of the rehabilitation program was fascinating. I never realized the process was so comprehensive and complex. "It must have been difficult to focus," I said. "I would think you had enough to do just dealing with the loss of your husband and son."

Faith gave me a wry grin. "On the contrary. The staff considered me to be their star pupil. The only class in which I did poorly was Mourning 101, which incidentally was actually part of the rehab program. The rehab program was a great distraction for me. By throwing myself into the process I was able to avoid dealing with my real loss. It was easier to accept that I no longer had the use of my legs than it was to face that I would never again see Danny and Zach."

Faith wiped her eyes with her sleeve. I felt bad that I had rekindled these painful memories. "Fortunately for me," she said, "there was a tenacious rehab counselor who wouldn't let me off the hook. After I mastered all of the physical skills and pretty much accommodated to the loss of my legs, I wanted to sign myself out of the program. The counselor, a feisty Irish woman who was even tinier than me, refused to certify that I had completed the program."

"What did you do?"

"My first response was to threaten to sue her and the hospital. Typical lawyer response. But she didn't back down and for some reason which I still don't understand, the hospital supported her. I actually think I would have won if it had gone to court."

"Judging from your performance with the detention center supervisor I think they would want to avoid facing you in a courtroom."

"Thanks. I'm a decent litigator, but I've lost my share of cases. Anyway I'm sure glad I didn't pursue this one. Once I threatened to sue them, the counselor offered a compromise: if I would spend a full week with her, she would sign my discharge, regardless of the outcome."

"That was quite an offer."

"In more ways than one. If it happened today, the managed care companies wouldn't have paid for more than three one-hour sessions."

"Jesus. Our system sure is screwed up. The Hammonds can't find help for their son without giving up custody. A person is supposed to work through the death of her husband and son in three sessions or less. The next thing you know we'll have same-day discharge for brain surgery."

"Frightening, isn't it? I was lucky in that respect. I'm certain I couldn't have accomplished what I did in a few hours. In fact, I spent the first day and a half glaring at my counselor, stubbornly refusing to talk. She finally gave me a pad of paper and asked me to write. She didn't care what I wrote as long as I filled the paper."

"Couldn't you avoid dealing with your loss just as easily with pen and paper?"

"I thought so. I started by making a grocery list. Then I wrote down the names of my favorite restaurants. I was obviously obsessed with food. Midway through my list I wrote down the name of a sushi place in the Village that Zach and I liked. Before I finished writing the name of the restaurant my hand started to tremble, my breathing became labored and I felt an enormous pressure building up inside me. Suddenly I was sobbing uncontrollably. The counselor let me cry for a moment. Then she knelt beside my chair, put her arms around me and held me until I was exhausted. We spent the next three days reliving the crash, allowing me to vent my feelings, and dealing with my anger, guilt, and sorrow. By the end of the week I was dealing with my grief in the same way I had confronted the other aspects of my rehabilitation program."

We were approaching the outskirts of Northampton and there were still a lot of questions I wanted to ask. I settled on the one I was most curious about: "Why did you stay in Northampton?"

Faith paused before responding. "I usually think of myself as a rational person. I've been trained in the rules of logic and I generally manage my life in an orderly and practical manner. The decision to live in Northampton is probably the most significant exception."

The car drifted onto the shoulder and Faith steered it back onto the road. "Sorry. I haven't talked about this for awhile. It tends to absorb my attention. Anyway, after my rehabilitation I returned to New York. Everyone was good to me. The law firm adapted my office and allowed me to modify my schedule to meet my needs. My friends and family were supportive. I moved into an accessible apartment and made special arrangements for transportation. Money wasn't a problem. Zach, in his typical fashion, had left me well provided for.

"Even with all of that support and convenience I felt dissatisfied. I kept thinking of Zach and Danny. Little things triggered intense memories. A birthday celebration at a favorite restaurant, buying Danny his first winter coat at Macy's, the Sunday comics. Even moving to another neighborhood didn't help."

"But why move here? I would think this area would stimulate painful memories."

"Strange, huh? It took me awhile to appreciate the perverse paradox of my decision. Several months after returning to New York I visited Northampton. Consciously I wanted to thank the rehab staff for the great job they had done. I now think a less conscious motive was at work. My best friend had volunteered to drive me here. When I got out of the car, I experienced an unusual sensation. For the first time since the accident I felt totally at ease. I had gone to college down the road at Mount Holyoke and had always liked this area. But my response that day was different. At first I thought I was grateful for all of the help I had received from the hospital staff. But it was more than that.

"It wasn't until the end of the weekend that I realized why I felt so good. In Northampton I felt close to Danny and Zach. Unlike my reaction in New York, where my memories only made me aware of the good things about them I had lost, my response here is not at all negative. I feel a strong connection to them, as if this is where their souls came to rest and by being here I could stay in touch with them."

The human mind constantly amazes me. Faith's memories of the happy life with her husband and son brought her only pain, while she was able to find solace and contentment at the site of their violent deaths.

Faith turned off Main Street and pulled up beside the building that housed her office. "I apologize for bending your ear. I don't usually unload on people like this."

"Getting run off the road tends to elicit unorthodox responses," I replied.

Faith frowned at me. "You're a fairly unorthodox private investigator. You sure don't talk like a private eye."

I hoped she didn't see me blushing. "I have a confession. I only moonlight as a private investigator. My day job is at Syracuse University. I'm a graduate student in psychology."

Faith covered her eyes with her hands. "Oh my God! You've probably been analyzing me all this time."

"No, I'm not that kind of psychologist. I'm in the social psychology doctoral program."

Recovering from her embarrassment, Faith chided me, "What other secrets are you keeping from me, Marty?"

"Only those that might provoke you to initiate legal action against me."

"No need to worry about that. Your pockets don't look very deep. Besides, I make it a practice not to sue my partner." She reached over and squeezed my hand.

This time I was certain she noticed the change in my complexion.

We put together a short to-do list. Faith was going to follow up with the district attorney to get a psychiatric evaluation for Tommy. She also agreed to do some research on how the Commonwealth handled emotionally disturbed kids who were accused of killing another person. My assignment was to visit Tommy's residential treatment center to find out more about him and the boy who had been murdered. We agreed to report back to each other late afternoon on the next day.

I got out of the car and watched Faith drive off. As I walked to the ice cream store to meet Ollie I wondered how Faith would be spending her evening.

CHAPTER EIGHT

Where's my mommy? I thought they were taking me home. But they took me here. It smells bad here. They took everything away. I want my mommy.

Bart's served upscale ice cream in a down-home ambiance. The walls were covered with an eclectic collection of cow art, all of which was for sale. The plastic tables were filled with young people munching on exotic flavors of ice cream and non-fat yogurt.

Ollie had not yet arrived, so I studied the wallboard menu while I waited for a table. At the table next to me a petite black woman and a large white woman were engaged in a heated debate about affirmative action. Without warning, the black woman slammed her coffee cup down, stood up, and stomped out of the store. The other woman sheepishly gathered her things and left quickly. Feeling like a participant in a game of musical chairs, I immediately slid into one of the empty chairs. The brief altercation between the two women made me think of the tension between Ollie and me. Not that our situation was likely to become explosive. I was too afraid of what she would do to me if she really lost her temper. I was beginning to understand what she had been saying to me. Our relationship wasn't working. Not just because I was looking for commitment and she wasn't. She was right that I could be persistent and would probably keep pursuing her until she knocked me on my butt. It was more basic than that. The things that had made our relationship so special, so exciting, were beginning to fade. The attraction and the passion were still there but it wasn't the same. And it wasn't just her. As much as I wanted to deny it the same spark wasn't there for me, either. As I was learning in graduate school it was great to have insight but what to do about it was another story. I decided to defer that challenge until later.

I turned my attention back to the wallboard menu. As I studied the extensive list of goodies I felt a gentle tap on my shoulder. I turned to see Ollie smiling down at me. Standing next to her was a tall, well-built blonde man who looked like he had just stepped out of Snow Country. He had the ruddy complexion of a person who spends a lot of time on the ski slopes and the wrinkles around his eyes were the only indication that he was not a young man.

"Hi, Marty," Ollie said cheerfully. "I'd like you to meet Lars Olafson. He was my sculpture professor at Smith. I bumped into him on campus and we had a nice chat about the good old days."

The green-eyed monster seized me by the throat. Why was she so cheerful? What did she mean, "bumped into him"? What exactly happened in the good old days? So much for insight. I swallowed hard, stood up and shook his hand. "Nice to meet you, Lars. Ollie has told me a lot about you."

I tried to avoid Ollie's quizzical look as I jockeyed desperately to establish a position of strength. Ollie had never told me about any of her professors, but I wanted to impress Lars with how well we communicated.

"Ollie has also told me about you," Lars replied. "She tells me you are a man of many talents."

"Oh," I said, wondering if "many talents" was a euphemism for "doesn't know what he wants to be when he grows up."

"Yes. She tells me you're working on a very important case while also finishing up your thesis."

"Ha," I chuckled. "Ollie tends to exaggerate. My work is not all that significant." My attempt to sound modest fell flat on its face. "Would you like to join us?" I said, once again lamely trying to establish where the real bond lay. "I hear the ice cream is pretty good."

Before Lars could reply, Ollie spoke. "Actually, there's a reception for the annual faculty art show. Lars is exhibiting some pieces and I want to see his work. I know you are not too interested in art so I thought we might meet you later for dinner. Oh, guess what, Marty. Remember how disappointed I was to find that Spoleto had closed? Actually it hasn't. It just moved to a larger location on the next block. How about we meet you there at seven-thirty?"

"I'd like to but I have some work to do on my case, so I think I'll pass. Have a good time."

"Are you sure?" Ollie asked.

"Yes. I've got a lot to do."

Ollie shrugged. "Okay. I'll catch up with you later. I made a reservation for us at a motel on the edge of town. It's not the Hotel Northampton, but it's clean." She reached into her purse and removed a small piece of paper which she handed to me. "Here's the address and phone number. The reservation's in your name."

Lars and I told each other how pleased we were to meet and then they left. I stared at the large menu board for a few minutes before deciding that I really didn't want ice cream.

I was surprised and disturbed by my reaction to Lars. Moments earlier I had acknowledged to myself that my relationship with Ollie was cooling not just because of her reluctance to make a commitment but also because my feelings were changing. Then she introduces me to her former professor and I react like a teenager whose girlfriend dumps him for his best friend. Very mature.

I wandered around town, looking into store windows and occasionally going into a shop. A salesperson in a well-stocked bookstore tried to engage me in a conversation about my reading interests but I was too distracted. After an hour of aimless walking I found myself in front of a restaurant with signs on its façade announcing that both traditional and exotic brews were served inside. I decided to interrupt my tour and stepped into the restaurant.

An oak bar ran the length of the front section of the restaurant. A few college-age men were seated at the bar, but the majority of its occupants were bikers in their thirties or forties and a few older men who appeared to have tenure at the establishment. The rear section of the restaurant had about a dozen tables covered with plastic cloths. Unlike the front of the restaurant, this room was inhabited exclusively by young men and women engaged in animated discussions while they ate oversized sandwiches and pasta dishes.

My choice was easy. I climbed up on a bar stool and ordered a pint of

Samuel Adams.

The other customers didn't take note of my presence, which was fine with me. I sipped my beer and felt sorry for myself. I finished my first beer in less than twenty minutes and ordered another pint. After I drank the second glass I considered ordering some food, but decided I wasn't hungry enough to eat.

I ordered another pint.

I'm not a big drinker. One beer is usually enough to give me a mild buzz. Occasionally I order a second beer, but I never drink more than half of it. So it is understandable that I was feeling light-headed after my third Samuel Adams.

My bladder also felt full so I asked the bartender where I could find the men's room. He pointed to a staircase and told me to turn right at the bottom. When I stood up I felt dizzy and had to wait for a moment until I felt steady enough to walk. I wobbled down the stairs and opened the first door I came to. I was relieved to see an unoccupied urinal and immediately unzipped my fly and stepped in front of it.

The room began to spin, so I leaned my forehead against the graffiti covered-wall. I felt a momentary twinge of anxiety about the germs I was picking up from the urinal wall, but my inebriation prevented me from holding any thought for more than a few seconds.

In a desperate attempt to bring the room under control I focused my attention on the creative scribbling on the walls. Aside from learning that Jennie's mother had a penchant for oversized male sexual organs and the telephone prefix five-eight-five was frequently associated with women who enjoyed oral sex, I wasn't able to glean much from the thoughtful prose left by former patrons.

Just as I felt that my bladder was going to burst the room stopped spinning. Feeling confident that I wouldn't soak my shoes, I gratefully began to relieve myself into the urinal, still supporting myself against the wall.

Worried that the stream I was producing might overflow the bowl I glanced down and was reassured to see that my concern was unjustified. I noticed a plastic drain guard at the bottom of the bowl. There was lettering on the drain guard and I had to squint to make out what it said.

Embossed on the plastic drain guard in small red letters was a simple, but authoritative command: Just Say No to Drugs.

I had seen that slogan before but never understood what I was supposed to do with it. Now, however, it took on new significance; the message seemed to be directed at me, personally. By guzzling three pints of beer I had crossed the line from social drinker to substance abuser. I was using alcohol to escape from reality, to avoid confronting my problem with Ollie. At that moment I was convinced that if I didn't repent immediately I would slide into a bottomless pit of self-destruction, imbibing beer and cheap whiskey to drown my sorrows until I ended up on skid row.

Armed with that insight, I was ready to take corrective action. I directed my attention to the drain guard, concentrating on its simple, but powerful message.

Then I cleared my throat and with as much conviction as I could muster, shouted "*No!*"

Nancy Reagan would have been proud of me.

As soon as I had spoken, the distinctive sound of a bowel erupting greeted me from the stall next to the urinal. This was followed by the voice of an older man, "You talkin' to me, sonny?"

"Pardon me," was my startled response.

"What's a matter, is ya deaf? I heard you say somethin' ta me and I wanna know what you was sayin'. As far as I can tell there's no one in this can but you and me. If ya got a problem wif me I wanna know what it is. If ya don't, ya oughta keep your thoughts to ya self."

"I'm sorry. I didn't know there was anyone else here."

"Yeah," the man in the stall said, releasing another round of gas. "Well watch ya'self. Jes cuz I'm sitttin' here on the throne don't mean I don't deserve some respect."

I quickly zipped up my fly and hurried out of the men's room.

While I was still a long way from being sober, the ground beneath my feet was stable and I was able to make my way upstairs without much difficulty. I had also regained some of my critical faculties. When the bartender asked if I wanted another drink I shook my head and asked instead for a cheeseburger, fries, and a cup of black coffee.

As I waited for my food I kept glancing at the stairs to see if my toilet mate would emerge. Several people went downstairs and returned but I didn't see anyone who might own that distinctive voice. I did, however, recognize a familiar face at the other end of the bar. Barry, the worker who had accompanied Faith and me when we visited Tommy at the detention center, was nursing a beer. He appeared to be alone.

I wanted to speak to him but decided it would be better to wait until some of the alcohol had worked its way out of my system. The bartender delivered my food and I wolfed it down. The cheeseburger was big and juicy; the fries were crisp and tasty. When I finished I felt almost normal. The bartender had just delivered my coffee when Barry stood up and started for the door.

"Hey, Barry, how you doing?" I said as he passed me.

He stopped and looked at me without any sign of recognition. Then his recent memory came on line and he smiled.

"You're the guy who came with the lady in the wheelchair. You were visiting that boy from the treatment center. Pretty spooky kid."

We shook hands and I invited him to join me. He hesitated briefly, then shrugged and sat down on the stool next to me.

"What are you drinking?" I asked. Ply them with alcohol and they'll tell you everything. Chapter Six, Fundamental principles for the professional investigator.

"I'll have a Coke," Barry answered.

So much for Chapter Six.

"How long have you worked at the detention center?" I asked.

"Almost four years. I work there part-time except summers. I'm getting my associates degree in criminal justice at the community college."

"You must see a lot of interesting kids."

"Yeah. Some real strange cases. I feel sorry for most of the kids, but every once in a while we get a hard-core psychopath who sends chills down my spine."

"How about Tommy? What do you think of him?"

Barry looked around before responding. "I'm not really supposed to talk about the kids outside of work. Confidentiality and all that good stuff. You know what I mean." I remained silent, borrowing this time from my friend Brad, who often shared with me the wisdom he gained from his clinical courses. Brad, whose memory-jogging ploy had failed so miserably with Ollie, told me that long silences often coax clients into speaking about things they are reluctant to reveal. I decided to give Brad another chance.

This time the technique worked. "I guess it's okay to talk to you," Barry said, lowering his voice. "You're authorized to visit him so I assume you have some official status."

Official status. I liked the sound of that.

"Tommy is one of the more unusual kids we've had," Barry continued. "He almost never talks. If you ask him if he wants milk for his cereal or if he needs to go to the bathroom he might say yes or no, but that's about it. Mostly he sits on his bed and rocks back and forth or paces from one side of his room to the other. In fact, that little scene with the lady in the wheelchair was the most active I've seen him since he came to the center."

"How is he with the other kids?"

"Can't really say. He's pretty much confined to the observation room. We've got strict instructions to limit his contact with the other residents. Guess they're afraid he might go off again."

"Again?" I asked, wondering if he was referring to the stabbing of the boy at the treatment center.

"Yeah. When he first came in there was an incident with one of the other kids. At that time they were letting him eat in the cafeteria. He was sitting at the table, eating his lunch, when he suddenly leaps across the table and starts choking the boy sitting across from him."

"Did the other kid do anything to provoke him?"

"I'm not sure. I wasn't working then, but one of the staff who was on duty thought he heard the other boy say something to Tommy."

"Do you remember the name of the other boy?"

Once again Barry hesitated, and again I assumed a position of therapeutic silence. This time Barry worked through his reluctance even more quickly. "Travis. Travis Jackson. I get him confused with another kid who came in at about the same time. Both of them have charges of aggravated assault. Funny thing is, Travis is a big boy. Looks like a tough kid. But I hear that it took two staff to pull Tommy off him."

I made a mental note to check on Travis Jackson.

Feeling good about my data-gathering achievement, I decided to probe some more. "What kind of place is the detention center?"

"It's okay for what it is. The kids who come to us aren't too happy about being there. Our main job is to keep them safe and secure. It's not like a hospital or a treatment center where they try to help kids. We baby-sit them while they're awaiting disposition."

"Must be frustrating."

"Sometimes. As I said before, most of the kids are okay. A lot of them come from screwed-up homes. They don't have any good role models. School is just another place that makes them feel bad about themselves. They get more attention for getting in trouble than for trying to be good."

"What do you get out of working at the center?"

Barry chuckled. "It pays my tuition. It also gets me some real-life material for my major. Lets me test the theories I learn in the classroom. Sometimes they don't hold up too well. And once in awhile I make a connection with a kid. I like to think I make a difference, at least with a few of them."

"I'm sure you do, Barry. You strike me as a caring person. What about the other staff?"

"They're mostly okay. Once in awhile we get someone who should be on the other side of the locked door, but that's the exception."

"Anyone like that working there now?"

"There's one guy on the evening shift that I have my doubts about. He's pretty mean to the kids. I've never seen him do anything abusive, but like I said, I have some doubts." Barry took a sip of his Coke and looked at me, anticipating my next question. "I don't feel right saying anything more about him."

"That's okay. I understand. How about the supervisor, Mr. Helfinger, what kind of guy is he?"

"He's harmless. Spends most of his time kissing the behinds of anyone who has influence on our budget or his performance evaluation. In one of my management courses we studied the different styles of organizational leadership: charismatic, visionary, et cetera. He doesn't fit any of those. He definitely subscribes to the philosophy that no good deed goes unpunished. He manages by the book but he never bothers to read the fine print. When in doubt, do nothing."

"Sounds like an inspiring leader."

"He's not that bad. At least he keeps the kids safe and well fed." Barry glanced at his watch. "I better be going. I've got a test tomorrow and I haven't even cracked the book."

I thanked him and shook his hand. He had a firm but not overbearing grip, consistent with my overall impression of him. My suspicious nature didn't allow me to completely rule him out of being involved with our road mishap, but I didn't have any tangible reason to suspect him.

I was deciding to order a second cup of coffee when I heard a familiar voice at the end of the bar. "Ya shoulda heard dis guy. He was shoutin' at me like I had done somethin' awful to his mother. I thought he was gonna climb inta the stall and beat the shit outta me."

I threw some money on the counter and hurried out of the restaurant.

Ollie was right. The motel she had chosen was not the Hotel Northampton. It was a one-story, wood-frame building which had not seen a paint brush in many years. The L-shaped structure looked like it had about twenty units. When I checked in the clerk asked whether I preferred deluxe, superior, or elegant accommodations.

I asked what the differences were and she patiently explained the distinctions in room size, bed type, and other accouterments. I was not impressed by the distinctions, but I'm not enamored with the current trend of using superlatives to describe ordinary commodities. I still become annoyed when my only choices for drink size are medium and large. I considered paying the extra two dollars for the superior room with the king size bed but chose instead to go with two double beds. Though my natural inclination is to save a few bucks whenever possible this decision was not based on economic considerations. Perhaps I was finally coming to grips with what was not going on between Ollie and me.

CHAPTER NINE

That big boy isn't nice. I'm trying to eat. He calls me bad names. Won't leave me alone. I get mad. Don't know what to do. He should leave me alone. I just want to eat lunch. I get really mad. I think I'm in trouble again.

By the time I settled into my standard room it was close to nine P.M. I began to read a detective novel I had bought at the second-hand bookstore, hoping to pick up some helpful hints. With one eye on the book and the other on the door I didn't make much progress. Finally I put down the book and took a shower.

The warm water helped my body, but didn't do much for my mind. My obsessive motor was in high gear. Had Ollie accidentally bumped into Lars or had she made plans to meet him? Had their relationship at Smith been strictly student-teacher or had it extended to extracurricular activities? How long could two people linger over dinner? Why was I thinking about this when I was fairly certain my relationship with Ollie was about to end?

I tried to shift my thoughts to Tommy Hammond and the events of the day, but that was equally nonproductive. I wondered if he knew what was happening to him. Though he appeared to be unresponsive to what was going on around him, I was convinced he must be terribly frightened. I thought about how we might get through to him, but couldn't think of anything that might work. In desperation I turned my attention to my thesis.

I couldn't get past the image of Professor Singleton hounding me for a completed copy of my results chapter.

Knowing I wouldn't be able to sleep I turned on the eleven o'clock news. I was always amused by how similar television newscasts were. The news seemed the same whether I was in Syracuse, Tampa or Toledo. Not just in content but also style. The female anchor with her perfect hair and clipped speech bantering with the casual but sincere male counterpart. I wondered if all newscasters were trained at the same school: the Sound Byte Institute or the Academy for the Advancement of Vacuous Broadcasting.

The news from Springfield that night included the usual array of fender benders, school budget impasses, and crimes against property and persons. There was one story, however, that caught my attention. An older woman was bringing suit against the Commonwealth of Massachusetts and the federal government for what she claimed to be an egregious violation of her constitutional rights as well as those of her family and ancestors. Her family had resided for many generations in a section of central Massachusetts known as the Swift River Valley. In the late 1930s, four towns were deliberately destroyed in order to create the Quabbin Reservoir, an enormous body of water that provides much of western Massachusetts with an excellent source of drinking water as well as recreational opportunities.

The woman suing the government claimed that the destruction of Enfield, the town in which her family resided, had been executed with neither due process not adequate regard for the property rights of the valley's inhabitants. She wanted the government to restore the valley to its original condition or pay each descendant of the four towns fifty million dollars to compensate for physical and psychological hardship.

Her claim gave new meaning to the term class action suit.

The attorney for the Commonwealth dismissed her charges as unfounded and preposterous. He said that the probability of her succeeding was about the same as those of a Red Sox fan nominating George Steinbrenner for sainthood.

The last clip of the story showed the woman, a soft-spoken, well-dressed silver-haired matron standing in front of the American flag. In one hand she held a replica of the Constitution of the United States. A copy of the New Testament was clasped in her other hand. Her last words on camera were, "The government may have might, but we have right on our side."

93

I wished her luck, turned off the television and tried to fall asleep.

Two hours later I lay in bed, no closer to sleep than I had been earlier. When the phone rang I picked it up before the second ring. "Hi, it's Ollie. I hope I didn't disturb you."

Disturb me, yes. Wake me, no. "What time is it?" I asked, trying to sound nonchalant.

"Uh, it's almost one-thirty. I'm sorry I didn't call earlier. We ran into some other professors I studied with and went to have coffee at my art history teacher's home."

More of that bumping and running into stuff. "That's nice. Did they whip out the slide projector and show some pictures of Mesopotamian folk art?"

"You're angry, aren't you?"

I hesitated briefly. Did I want to get into this at one-thirty in the morning? I was angry. But at least as much at myself as with her. Why couldn't I deal directly with what was happening between us? "I expected you to be back earlier. I thought we were going to spend some time together, try to work things out."

"You're right. I didn't expect to run into Lars. I guess at some level I was grateful for the distraction. I've been so confused about our relationship."

Distraction. Is that what Lars was? Television was a distraction, a mosquito buzzing in your ear was a distraction. I couldn't picture Lars as a distraction. A Norse god, maybe; a sex object, perhaps; but a distraction, not likely. Slow down, jerk, I thought. If anyone's getting distracted it's me. "Where are you now?"

"I'm at Lars' studio. He's showing me some of his recent work."

His etchings, no doubt. It was no use. My attempts at rational thinking were doomed to failure. If I didn't deal with what was really happening soon I would drive myself and Ollie over the edge. I took a deep breath before I speaking. "I . . . I don't know what to say," I began. "Seeing you with Lars . . . I guess it threw me for a loop. I was feeling shaky about our relationship already and the shock of seeing you reacting with such excitement to this tall, handsome man. I know that the real issue is what's going on between you and me, not with Lars. And I also realize that it's not just your problem, that I'm as responsible if not more so for the problems in our relationship." My throat began to tighten and my eyes swelled. "I'm afraid of losing you, Ollie. At the same time I know that you're right, that our relationship isn't what it was or what either of us wanted it to be. I'm just having trouble dealing that. Nothing I do helps. I see myself acting like an asshole but I can't seem to do anything about it."

There was a painful silence. I prayed that she would say something. I had revealed more than I had intended.

"Thank you," she whispered.

"Are you coming to the motel?" I asked with some trepidation.

"No. I'm going to stay at Lars' place tonight. He has an extra room."

"Oh, I see."

At the other end of the line Ollie was making unusual sounds. At first I couldn't tell if they were sad or happy noises. But as the sounds became louder, there was no longer any doubt: Ollie was laughing. Not just a polite party-conversation chuckle. This was a full-bodied belly laugh.

"What the hell is so funny?" I asked indignantly.

"I know what you're thinking. You've got such a typical male mind."

"But . . ."

"Take it easy. You don't have anything to worry about. I promise to be a good girl."

"It's not you I'm concerned about."

"As I said, you have nothing to worry about."

"Yeah, okay."

"You're really worried about Lars, aren't you?"

Her direct confrontation made me feel a little foolish. "I guess so."

"Well, you don't have to be."

"Easy for you to say."

"Jesus, Marty. Do I have to spell it out for you? Lars isn't going to ravage me because he isn't interested in me that way. Lars is gay."

Now I felt even more foolish.

What vain creatures we of the male species are.

We agreed to meet in town for lunch the next day. Sensing that I might need an extra measure of reassurance, she even gave me Lars' home and studio telephone numbers in case I wanted to reach her.

I must have fallen asleep within moments of putting down the phone.

When I awoke at eight, slightly hung over, the light next to the bed was still on. I took a quick shower and got dressed. Remembering that the motel offered a free continental breakfast I stopped at the reception area, picked up a couple of donuts and a cup of bitter coffee.

Then I set out to visit the Possum Ridge School, hoping my luck would soon change.

CHAPTER TEN

*They keep talking about Kevin. I don't like Kevin. He makes
me mad. He always makes fun of me. Why doesn't he leave
me alone? I don't bother him. He keeps picking on me. For no
reason. He's going to be sorry if he doesn't stop.*

Located fifteen miles to the north and east of Northampton,
Possum Ridge made a better first impression than the detention
center. As I approached the school, the name conjured up images
of kids hanging by their feet from specially designed racks designed to
correct their chemical imbalance. I was pleasantly surprised to find a
cluster of attractive modern cedar shingle buildings. There were several
well-equipped-playing fields, one of which had a ropes course. There was
a chain-link fence encircling one of the buildings. The fence did not have
barbed wire at the top.

I pulled into the parking lot and followed the signs that directed
visitors to report to a large building at the front of the complex. The
receptionist greeted me warmly, another contrast to the detention center,
and asked me who I wanted to see. I explained the purpose of my visit
and she asked me to have a seat while she located someone to help me.

In less than two minutes a tall, middle-aged woman approached me
and held out her hand. "Hello, Mr. Fenton. I'm Ms. Harrington. I'm Dr.
Prosic's assistant. He's meeting with a family now and asked me to help
you."

She led me down a corridor of offices to a small, tastefully furnished
room. On our way we passed a door with a large sign indicating that
Harold P. Prosic, Ph.D. was the director of the school, sparing me the
embarrassment of asking who Dr. Prosic was.

Ms. Harrington offered me a cup of coffee, which I gratefully accepted. While I sipped the coffee, which was significantly better than the cup I had picked up at the motel, she studied the court order I had given to her. When she was finished she excused herself, telling me she would be back in a moment.

True to her word she returned shortly and asked me to come with her. We stopped in front of the door with Dr. Prosic's name on it and she knocked twice.

"Please come in." The voice on the other side of the door was deep and pleasant. The room we entered was much larger than Ms. Harrington's but just as nicely appointed. Seated behind a large walnut desk in the center of the office was an enormous doe-eyed man. He wore a charcoal pinstripe suit with a white shirt and gray and red striped tie. Besides his size—he must have weighed close to three hundred fifty pounds—his most noticeable feature was his hair. Combed in a style popular in the nineteen fifties, his thick brown hair was shaped into a large pompadour in front, followed by a series of smaller waves, all of which were held in place by a quantity of grease sufficient to lubricate a mid-size automobile.

"You've come a long way to visit us," the man behind the desk said. "I trust you had a good journey."

"I did," I responded as I reached across the desk to shake his hand. He did not make any effort to rise.

"I'm Harold Prosic and this is my trusted assistant, Gloria Harrington. It's our job to keep this school operating in a compassionate, professional, and efficient manner. Not an easy task, especially these days. Between the budget crises and managed care we can barely afford the chewing gum and spit needed to hold the place together. Last year we ran a two-hundred-thousand-dollar deficit, the first negative balance we've had in over twenty-six years of operation."

That's nice, I thought. But why is he telling me this?

As if she was reading my mind, Harrington said. "But you didn't come here to listen to our woes. How can we help you?"

I explained that the Hammonds had hired me to find out what was happening with Tommy. Because they had transferred custody of Tommy to the Department of Social Services they were having difficulty getting access to information about their son.

Prosic nodded sympathetically. "An unfortunate situation," he said. "In many ways I empathize with the Hammonds' plight. The custody transfer requirement is archaic and cruel. Imagine having to give up the basic rights of parenthood to get help for your child. I know it's only supposed to be a formality, but as you can see, many social service agencies interpret the policy literally. Unfortunately it's the only way to get funding for kids like Tommy. We don't have much choice." He looked at Ms. Harrington briefly, then turned his attention to the ceiling.

"Some states have adopted legislation prohibiting the custody transfer practice," Ms. Harrington said. "And there's a bill in Congress that would make it illegal for any state or locality to require parents to relinquish custody in order to receive services."

"Until then, I guess we have to live with it," Prosic said, returning to the conversation. "Right now, that's not the worst of our worries. Kevin's death was devastating. The children are terribly disturbed, the staff are beside themselves, and the families of our residents are afraid for the safety of their young ones. Several families have already withdrawn their children."

"As if that's not bad enough," Harrington added, "the police and the regulatory agencies have been here constantly, asking questions, reviewing records. It's been quite disruptive to our program."

"Speaking of the program," I said, trying to steer the conversation back to Tommy. "Can you tell me anything about how he was doing while he was here?"

Prosic glanced at his assistant before responding. "Tommy is an extremely troubled boy. His problems are long-standing and have not proven to be amenable to traditional treatment. From what we can gather he comes from a relatively caring and nurturing home so it is unlikely that his disturbance was environmentally induced. We struggled with his diagnosis for a long time. Initially we thought he might suffer from pervasive developmental delay or even autism. We're now fairly certain that Tommy has schizophrenia, though for obvious reasons we're reluctant to make that diagnosis official. Most people with schizophrenia show signs of deterioration in early adulthood. Some have onset in their late teen years, but only a small percentage become ill before that. We think Tommy may be one of those rare exceptions."

"What was he like while he was here?" I asked.

I thought I saw Harrington nod at Prosic. "He was mostly quiet and withdrawn," Prosic said. He pulled himself forward so he could rest his elbows on the desk. Clasping his hands together, he continued his description of Tommy's behavior. "Most of the time he stayed to himself. There were a couple of staff who related well to him and sometimes he tried to play with the younger kids. But they didn't really like having him around. About the only area he excelled in was math. He's a bright boy and when he is able to focus he does quite well."

"That figures," I said.

"What do you mean?" Prosic asked, looking puzzled.

"Tommy's father's an engineer."

Prosic glanced at Harrington, looking for guidance. She ignored him, turning toward me, instead. "There was one other activity he liked. Occasionally the dietitian would bring him back to the kitchen to bake. They would make bread or cookies. Sometimes they would bake a cake from scratch. Tommy really enjoyed cooking. Once I even caught him grinning at a chocolate layer cake he and the dietitian had baked. "

I recalled the photo of Tommy in his high chair, his cake-smeared face smiling at me. Having seen Tommy curled up on his mattress yesterday, I had difficulty imagining him grinning now. "What did he do with the food? Did he eat it himself or did he share it with the other kids?"

Harrington shrugged. "I don't know. I haven't seen him interact with other kids. But I'm not sure. I'll ask Mrs. Macovey, the dietitian."

Once again I caught Prosic staring up at the ceiling, his lips moving. Either I was boring him or Dr. Prosic was engaged in another conversation with someone not visible to me. I knew my repartee was not terribly scintillating, but I didn't think I was that dull.

Sensing that the discussion was waning, Harrington asked, "Is there anything else you would like to ask?"

"Not at the moment. Perhaps I can speak to some of the staff on Tommy's unit?"

My question brought Prosic back to our plane. "No problem. We can arrange that. Gloria will walk you over there. Be sure to speak to Mr. Washington. He knew Tommy as well as anyone. Wouldn't you agree, Gloria?"

Gloria did not seem thrilled by his suggestion, but not having any better ideas, she agreed to escort me to Tommy's former unit. I shook hands with Prosic—again he did not rise -and thanked him for his help.

Harrington did not speak until we had left the administration building. "Dr. Prosic is not always like this. He's under a lot of pressure. Last year for the first time the center ran a deficit. Managed care is killing us."

Not being a clinician I'm reluctant to make judgments about people's mental status, but I was fairly confident that Dr. Prosic's behavior was more than just a situational response to changing trends in mental health care funding. Though I was curious about Prosic's unusual mannerisms I was more interested in learning more about Tommy Hammond. Although the evidence was stacked against him, I wasn't ready to accept the conclusion that Tommy had killed Kevin. There was no question that Tommy was capable of violence. His parents' accounts of his explosive behavior at home and in school, and the incident at the detention center left little room for doubt that Tommy would inflict harm on others, often without much obvious provocation. But the pattern of his aggression was fairly consistent. He struck out with his hands and feet, punching, choking, kicking. Not once had he used a stick or a tool or a knife.

As a legal defense my argument was rather weak. I didn't know about all of Tommy's aggressive acts. He might have used some sort of instrument to hurt someone in the past. That was one of the things I wanted to find out during my visit to Possum Ridge. Even if I found out that he had resorted to using something other than his hands and feet to strike out at others, there were still some important unanswered questions, the most significant being: What could have happened to provoke Tommy Hammond to plunge a knife into Kevin Landry's chest?

I filed away my curiosity about Harold Prosic and focused my attention on Tommy Hammond.

"Did Tommy spend much time with Kevin?"

"Not really," Harrington replied. "They lived in the same cottage but didn't share any interests. In fact, I don't think you could find two boys at Possum Ridge who were more dissimilar. Kevin was a real people person. If he wasn't playing basketball or engrossed in a card game he was recounting stories about his life before coming to Possum Ridge.

I even caught him flirting with one of the girls a few times. He was a handsome boy with a good sense of humor. Except for his bravado, which occasionally got on my nerves, he was a nice kid. You've met Tommy, so I don't think I need to spell out the contrast."

We were crossing a well-equipped playing field with a softball diamond and soccer goal at the far end and a playground next a small one story building at the other end. A half dozen teenage boys were playing touch football on the open field while two girls on the swing set laughed heartily as they propelled themselves skyward. Two young adults and an obese child sat on a bench watching the others play. It seemed so normal; a schoolyard, a neighborhood playground.

"What was Kevin here for? I asked."

Harrington hesitated before responding. "I'm not sure the rules of confidentiality allow you access to that information."

"What do you mean, confidentiality? Kevin's dead. I don't think he's going to mind if you tell me the reason he was sent to your school. Besides, I'm sure the district attorney has his entire case record. It's not fair to give information to one side, but not the other."

"It's different," Harrington responded defensively. "The district attorney has legal standing. You're just a private investigator. You're not even a lawyer."

"Thanks for the compliment. But I think you're nit-picking. Tommy's lawyer and I have divided up the investigation. She asked me to visit the school while she checked with the court."

Red splotch marks appeared on Harrington's throat. She did not seem to be enjoying our conversation. "You may have a point, Mr. Fenton. However, I'm not comfortable sharing that information without first checking with our legal counsel."

I wasn't comfortable with her *not* sharing the information but didn't think there was much I could do at that moment to expand my comfort zone. "When can you check with your counsel?" I asked, making no attempt to conceal my frustration.

"I'll make a call while you're visiting the unit. Hopefully Mr. Fiske's not in court."

By this time we were at the entrance of the small building adjacent to the playground. A small sign over the door let us know that we were entering the Maple Unit which housed the Early Adolescent Intermediate Program. I wondered whether intermediate referred to the size of the children, the severity of their problems, or the length of their tenure at the school. Given the residual tension that lingered from my last question I decided to wait for a better moment to clarify what the term meant.

"This is the day room," Harrington said as we stepped into a large, brightly painted room. A pair of comfortable-looking sofas faced a television that was set inside a closet behind a glass door. There were a couple of round game tables with attached benches, more attractive but functionally similar to those I had seen at the detention center, several wood-frame easy chairs with plaid cushions and a ping pong table that was taking a pounding from two large boys who were long on power and short on finesse.

There were about a dozen people in the room. A few watched TV, several sat at one of the tables playing cards, a couple played Nintendo, and the rest sat alone either reading or napping.

A small boy who had been watching TV jumped up as soon as we entered the room and ran to us. He was a pale, thin youngster with dark brown hair that looked as if it had been styled by a proponent of the bowl-on-head school of tonsorial science. With his oversized green and red checked shirt and baggy blue and yellow striped pants, he either was a mini clone of Professor Singleton or was a sure bet for a supporting role in the musical *Oliver*.

"Miss Harrington," he said, reaching up and pulling on her sleeve. "Am I going on pass this weekend? Can I visit my sister? How about I stay with my foster parents?" His voice was loud and shrill but nobody paid attention to him.

Harrington gently removed his hand from her arm. "What did I tell you, Ricky?" This was obviously a conversation that the two of them had engaged in numerous times, but there was no trace of impatience in her voice. She stood there holding Ricky's hand in hers, waiting for him to respond.

When Ricky saw that she was not going to say anything, he said, "I don't know. I can't remember."

Harrington patted his hand. "I told you that your case worker is working on getting you a new placement. When she gets one she will let you know. Then you can go on a pass. And you know why you can't visit your sister. Last time you went to her house you smashed your plate on the floor when she said you couldn't have a third helping of spaghetti. Then you hit her husband on the arm when he tried to help you settle down. I don't think you'll be visiting you sister in the near future."

Sensing that this line of inquiry wasn't going anywhere, Ricky turned his attention to me. "Are you my new case worker? Have you found me a new foster home yet?"

"No, Ricky, this isn't your new case worker," Harrington said before I could respond. "This is Mr. Fenton. He's visiting Possum Ridge today."

"You're not here for me?" Ricky asked.

As soon as I shook my head, Ricky snatched his hand away from Ms. Harrington and ran back to the TV set.

I began to ask why Ricky was at Possum Ridge, but caught myself midway through the question. Ms. Harrington wrinkled her brow into a frown, then broke out into a grin.

"Almost got me that time," she said.

"I'm sorry. I really don't have any reason to know Ricky's life story."

"That's okay. Some of these kids are pretty heart-wrenching. It's hard not to wonder how they ended up like this. Besides, curiosity is an essential prerequisite for being a private investigator. I'd be surprised if you didn't ask questions."

At that moment there was a commotion at the ping pong table. Two large boys, having grown tired of venting their frustration on the ball, were now directing their hostility toward each other. They began by shouting across the table, each accusing the other of cheating. When the allegations shifted from unsportsmanlike conduct to their mothers' sexual preferences, the boys moved from behind the security of the ping pong table and confronted each other nose-to-nose. Just as it looked as if the conflict threatened to become physical, a thin black man stepped between them.

I had noticed the man when we first entered the day room. He was constantly in motion. He moved from group to group, head bobbing, hands waving, bouncing on his toes as he moved around the room, stopping just long enough to give a thumbs-up sign of encouragement or pat someone on the shoulder.

At first, I thought he was one of the kids. He was smaller than several of the older boys and his shirt and jeans, shaved head, and near manic pace gave him the appearance of a hyperactive, easily distractible adolescent.

"Watch this," Harrington whispered to me as the small black man inserted himself between the two angry boys. I wasn't sure what she wanted me to watch. The only image that came to mind was a fluttering bird being crushed by an enormous vise. It was not a pretty image.

When the boys began to shout at each other, all activity in the room came to a halt. A couple of staff members moved the other children away from the confrontation. The tension in the room was palpable as everyone focused on the three people standing by the ping pong table.

The first thing the slim black man did was to turn to the larger boy, rise up on his toes and whisper something into his ear. I couldn't hear what he said, but was relieved when the boy took a couple of steps backward. He continued to glare at the other boy but stopped shouting at him.

Next, the man turned to the other boy, who stood in a crouch, ping pong paddle clutched in his fist. His menacing stance and snarling mouth made him look like a vicious dog.

"Let me at him," the boy in the crouch said. "Let me at the son of a bitch. I'll rip his fucking head off."

"You don't have to do this, Mickey," the man said softly. He was standing less than a foot from the boy, arms at his side. It took a few seconds for me to realize that all of his hyperactive behavior, the bobbing and bouncing, the wild hand gestures, had stopped. He stood perfectly still, looking up into Mickey's eyes, waiting for a response.

"I'll kill the bastard," Mickey said, still furious.

"And where will that get you? You're almost sixteen. Next time you go before the judge it won't be in kiddy court. You'll do hard time, a lot of hard time. You've been working so hard. You earn one more level and you'll be able to go on a weekend pass. Another couple months and you'll be out of here. Use your strategy, man. Make it work for you."

Mickey shifted his feet. I held my breath. The slim black man didn't move a muscle. "The fucker cheated," Mickey shouted. "Not just that, he called my momma a rotten name. I can't let the prick get away with that. He . . . he's gone too far this time."

At the other end of the room a thin boy with long scraggly hair began to scream hysterically. Two staff standing near the boy conferred briefly and then one of them took the boy by his hand and escorted him out of the day room.

None of the people at the ping pong table seemed to notice.

The black man shook his head slowly and said, "It's only a ping pong game, Mickey. Are you willing to throw it all away for a crummy ping pong game?" He paused for a few seconds, keeping his gaze on Mickey's face. "Besides," he continued, "you're a lousy ping pong player. You're good at a lot of things. There isn't a better fullback in the school and with a little practice you'll be a real bad bass guitarist. But let's face it, you couldn't beat Eric at ping pong even if he cheated in your favor."

A couple of the younger kids giggled, but when Mickey looked in their direction, they became silent. The taller boy at the ping pong table, whom I assumed was Eric, shrugged self-consciously. Mickey shifted the ping pong paddle to his other hand.

The slender man slowly moved his right head and scratched his shaved head. "What's it going to be? You going to work for yourself or back yourself into the toilet? Your choice, man, I can't make it for you."

Mickey shuffled his feet slightly before responding. "Yeah, but what about my momma? I can't let him say them things about her. It ain't respectful."

For the first time, the small man broke eye contact with Mickey. Taking a few steps backward, he stopped next to Eric. He reached up and placed his hand firmly on the back of the taller boy's neck. He looked at each of the boys several times before speaking. "Eric is one fine ping pong player," he said showing him a wide grin. "But he isn't too good at expressing himself. Now, when he said your mother was a rotten you-know-what, I'm pretty sure he was trying to tell you that your momma is a good lady and she could never be a good you-know-what. In fact, she would make a rotten you-know-what. Isn't that right, Eric?"

It took Eric a few seconds to figure out what the man standing next to him was saying, but he finally understood and nodded. He was obviously reluctant to tangle with Mickey and the absurd logic of the black man's explanation provided him with a good opportunity to save face.

Mickey, on the other hand, did not seem as ready to call it quits. The slender man did not give him a chance to weigh his alternatives. He stepped toward the young man, with the same bounce he had shown before the confrontation, plucked the paddles from his hand, and threw his arm around Mickey's shoulders. "How about we toss a football? I understand the older adolescent unit wants to challenge us to a game of flag football and we better be ready to whip their butts."

At that point, Mickey didn't seem to have much choice. "I guess so," he said, nodding.

"Okay, the party's over," the slender man said. "Eric, you go with Ms. Caldwell and have a little talk about setting up your peers. The rest of you get ready for school." Catching the successful negotiator's attention, Ms. Harrington formed her thumb and forefinger into a circle and raised it to him in a signal of approval. Then she motioned him to join us. He whispered something in Mickey's ear. Mickey grinned and took a seat at the table. The small man with the shaved head skipped across the room to us.

"Nice work, Bernard," the assistant director said, patting him on the shoulders. "I wish we could bottle your skills and serve it in the staff cafeteria."

Bernard shrugged. "It's nothing more than common sense. These kids look and act tough, but mostly they're scared and hurt. Like wounded animals. If you corner them they're going to attack. Give them a little space and some respect and they'll be okay." I noted that Bernard didn't look at Gloria Harrington as he spoke. He kept glancing over his shoulder, looking at the children.

"I wish it were as simple as you make it sound," Harrington said. "Maybe you can put together an in-service training program for unit staff. In the meantime, I'd like you to meet Mr. Fenton. He has some questions about Tommy Hammond and I thought you would be a good person for him to speak with. Mr. Fenton, this is Bernard Washington, program coordinator for the early adolescent unit. Mr. Fenton is a private investigator. He's been hired by Tommy's parents to find out more about Tommy's involvement in the . . . terrible incident the other night. Do you think you could spend a few minutes with him?"

Bernard nodded as he held out his hand. He looked directly into my eyes as we shook hands. He had a firm grip.

"I have a quality improvement meeting in a few minutes," Harrington said. "I think Mr. Fenton should also speak to Dr. Clover, Tommy's therapist. Would you mind dropping him off at her office when you're done? I'll call her so she'll know you're coming."

As soon as Harrington left, Bernard turned to the boy in the chair and said, "I hope you have some spring in your legs, Mickey. My arm's feelin' real strong."

"No problem, Mr. Washington," the boy said, pulling a baseball cap from his pocket as he walked toward us. "No offense, but I haven't seen you throw a ball that I couldn't catch." He put the cap on his head with the peak facing backward. "Except the one's that slipped out of your hand when you try to do your Tom Brady windup."

Bernard gave the boy a playful punch on the arm and reached up to put his arm around his shoulders. "Mickey, this is Mr. Fenton. He's a scout for the Chicago Bears. They're looking for a new quarterback and they've narrowed their choices down to two guys: Vince Young and me. If you make me look good I might take you along."

"Yeah, right," Mickey said, adjusting his cap as he looked at me curiously.

Once we were outside Bernard asked Mickey to retrieve the football, which was at the far end of the playing field. "You don't mind if we talk while I play catch with him, do you?" he said as Mickey ran to get the ball. It sounded more like a statement than a question.

"No problem. I appreciate you giving me some time. I can see that you're busy. Incidentally, I was really impressed by how you handled that situation on the unit. If you don't get recruited by the Bears you might consider a career in the diplomatic corps. They could use someone with your skills in the Middle East."

Bernard smiled, showing a large gold-capped tooth. "Like I said before, it's nothing but common sense." He caught the ball Mickey had tossed to him and directed the large boy to run a down and out pattern. He threw a line-drive pass that Mickey grabbed with two hands and pulled into his chest. The impact of the ball made me wince but the boy didn't flinch. "Nice catch," Bernard shouted. "Next one won't be so soft." Bernard turned to me and said, "I don't know what anyone else has told you, but there's no way Tommy could have killed Kevin."

It took a few seconds for his words to register. This was the first time since the Hammonds had hired me that someone had directly challenged the allegation that Tommy was responsible for Kevin's death. Not that I had accepted that the charges were valid. The story was sketchy; the evidence too circumstantial. Doubt had quietly gnawed at the back of my mind.

But I was hard-pressed to come up with an alternative explanation. That was what I hoped to find on my visit to Possum Ridge.

Bernard's simple declaration had triggered a faint pulse of encouragement within me. I fought back my urge to allow it premature expression.

"What makes you say that?" I asked, trying to keep the excitement out of my voice.

Bernard studied my face briefly before responding.

"Tommy Hammond is one whacked-out kid. If he's lucid more than ten minutes in a shift we consider it a good day. And no one will dispute that he can be violent. I've seen him go through a room like a tornado, smashing everything in his path. I've also seen him punch out a kid twice his size. But this incident, Kevin's murder, isn't consistent with Tommy's M.O."

"How so?"

"Two things don't fit. First, there's no reason Tommy would be in Kevin's room. They didn't have anything in common; they certainly weren't friends. And Tommy's not a wanderer. He left his room when staff told him: to go to the cafeteria, to school, even the day room. Otherwise he was content to stay in his room."

"What if someone lured him out? Isn't there something he liked that one of the kids might have promised to give him? Candy, games, something like that."

"Not likely. Tommy's a pretty self-contained kid. He has a few objects he's attached to: an iPod, a Game Boy, some comic books. He's not interested in anything that isn't part of his small collection. As far as food, he eats when he's told. He doesn't have the same attraction to food the other kids do."

"Maybe Kevin provoked him."

Bernard shook his head. He picked up the football and threw a long pass that Mickey couldn't quite catch up to. "Sorry Mick," he shouted,

"My bad." Turning back to me he said, "That kid's got real potential, not just in football. Comes from a lousy home. Father beat the shit out of him every time he sneezed. His mother drank herself to death. Her way of coping, I guess. Considering where he came from, Mickey could be doing a lot worse. He's got a good heart and excellent mechanical aptitude. If he can build up some self-confidence and get control of his temper he'll be okay."

Apparently Bernard didn't share Ms. Harrington's concern for confidentiality. On the other hand, he certainly seemed to care a lot about the kids.

"Why are you so confident Kevin didn't provoke Tommy?" I asked.

"Kevin was a street-wise kid. He had his fair share of fights and he wasn't above taking risks. He had a long record of juvenile offenses: shoplifting, breaking and entering, that kind of thing. He also was smart enough to know when to draw the line. He'd seen Tommy go off and I'm confident he didn't want any part of that action. Kevin was a survivor." As soon as the words were out of his mouth, Bernard closed his eyes and slapped himself on the head. "Bad choice of words. You know what I mean, though."

I nodded sympathetically. "Could one of the other kids—how did you say it back there in the day room—set up Kevin?"

"No way"

"How can you be so sure?"

"Because of the other reasons Tommy couldn't have killed Kevin. All of the damage Tommy did, whether to people or property, he did with his hands or his feet and occasionally his head. He never used objects when he acted out. I'm not sure why. It certainly didn't have anything to do with an aversion to blood and gore. I once saw Tommy nearly gouge out the eye of a new kid who had baited him in order to impress the older boys. I only know that his choice of weapons is limited to his own body parts."

I tucked this information away in my memory bank. It confirmed my earlier observation and might prove to be useful in my future inquiries.

Mickey tossed the ball in and Bernard handed it to me. "Why don't you throw a few. My arm is getting tired." I rolled the ball in my hands. It had been a long time since I had played football, at least five or six years.

The ball looked awfully big.

My testosterone flowing, I directed Mickey to go deep. I waited a few seconds, allowing him to sprint twenty to twenty-five yards down field. Then I wound up and threw the ball as hard as I could.

The ball came off my fingertips and headed skyward. I was hoping for one of those high arching spirals, a Hail Mary pass that the receiver leaps for in the end zone and snares with his finger tips. Instead the ball began to wobble as soon as it left my hand. It had height, but that was all. I watched the ball spin out of control as it ascended, hoping it would drop quickly to the ground and end my embarrassment. It seemed to linger interminably at its apex before falling to the ground like an inebriated man rolling down a hill.

Seeing that the ball was going to fall far short of its mark, Mickey made a valiant effort to minimize my embarrassment. He stopped in his tracks, spun around and raced toward the plunging missile. Just as the ball was about the hit the ground, Mickey dove horizontally and grabbed the pigskin with his large hands.

"Great job," Bernard shouted as Mickey shook the dust from his clothes. Then he turned to me with a grin and asked, "Been awhile since you played?"

I didn't bother to respond.

Bernard spared me further humiliation by telling Mickey to do five laps. We walked to the sideline and sat on a bench while the large boy circled the field. We talked about Possum Ridge, how kids came to be residents of the school, why Bernard chose to work there. I was impressed with his insight and intelligence, but even more so with his dedication to the kids. He told me he had a master's degree in social work and had turned down a number of administrative positions that paid considerably more and required less effort than his position as program coordinator. His day began at seven-thirty in the morning and usually ended between seven and eight in the evening. Unlike other coordinators he preferred to spend most of his time with the children rather than sitting in front of a computer, checking elaborate activity and work schedules.

He hesitated when I asked his opinion of Possum Ridge. His response, when it came, was succinct: Possum Ridge was a good place. It had been better and would become worse unless some changes were made soon.

111

I asked him to elaborate but he declined. I decided not to press him on that subject.

Bernard was not as reserved when he discussed the children and the reasons they were sent to Possum Ridge. "They have a lot of fancy labels for these kids," he said, standing up and beginning to pace in front of the bench. "Emotionally disturbed, behaviorally disordered, mentally ill. They sound good but they don't tell the real story. Sure these kids have problems. They wouldn't be here if they didn't. Some of them, like Mickey, drew the short straw in the family lottery. If Mickey had a decent family he would have done fine. Then there's kids like Tommy Hammond. He's a real sick boy. I don't know if its genetic or he picked up some virus when he was a baby. I only know his brain isn't firing on all cylinders. That's technical talk, incidentally."

"So you don't think Tommy's problems could have been caused by the way his parents treated him?"

"Hell, no. Tommy could have been raised by the Walton family and he would still be as screwed up as he is today." He had accelerated his pacing, walking from one end of the bench to the other, turning around and retracing his steps.

"So what can a place like Possum Ridge do? I know there are a lot of medications for psychiatric problems: thorazine, lithium, Prozac. But as far as I know they just control symptoms. They haven't found any cures, have they?"

"Not that I know of. But that's no excuse. They could do a lot better with what they have."

He was losing me. "Who are 'they' and what could they do better with?"

Bernard stopped and gave me a bewildered look. Then he threw his head back and laughed. "I'm sorry. I get carried away when I talk about the kids. It also doesn't help that I'm attention deficit disordered. Of course that's just another one of those half-truth labels, but in my case it at least has some validity. When it comes to staying focused on a subject I have the attention span of a two-year-old."

"And you were saying?" I said, unable to resist the opening.

"Touché," he said, pointing at me. "What I was trying to say is that the kids aren't sent to Possum Ridge because of their diagnosis. They end up here because their communities and the agencies that are supposed to take care of them have given up on them. The schools, the courts, social services, community mental health. They're supposed to help kids and their families, and often they do. There are some kids, however, those who come to Possum Ridge—or land in correction facilities—who they don't help. Either the kids' problems are too tough, or they require more resources than the agencies are willing to commit. Even worse, there are kids who make the agencies and communities uncomfortable. At some point the powers-that-be give up and decide to cut their losses. The message goes out: get rid of this kid."

"You make it sound like a conspiracy," I said, taken aback by his strong view.

"It is, in a way. A conspiracy to deprive these kids of their rights as citizens of the community. They dress it up in fancy terms: treatment resistant, in need of a more protective setting, high risk. But it all boils down to one thing: We want this kid out of here. Someone a lot smarter than I am came up with a good name for these children: throwaway kids. I guess that makes us a landfill site for disposable children."

I watched Mickey begin his last lap and had a hard time imagining an entire community giving up on a boy whose principal liability was being born into an abusive family. And what about Tommy? I had seen how his parents agonized over their inability to care for him. Had all other sources of help really been exhausted or had the Syracuse children's service establishment decided that Tommy didn't fit into their game plan and banished him to the Pioneer Valley?

Was Bernard too cynical? Or was I blinded by my naive view of how the world worked?

CHAPTER ELEVEN

I don't like the medicine. It tastes bad. They tell me it will help me, but I don't believe them. They don't always tell the truth. My mommy says it isn't nice to lie. They laugh at me when I tell them. They don't like me.

D r. Clover's office was in the Elm Unit, a square cinder block structure at the far end of the playing field. The building's gray cement exterior stood in stark contrast to the attractive cedar buildings at the front of the property. Bernard explained that the Elm Unit housed children whose violent behavior had earned them admission to the juvenile corrections system. These youngsters were different than Mickey, whose aggressive behavior had not yet crossed the criminal threshold, at least in the eyes of the law. The kids in the Elm Unit had been adjudicated as delinquents by a juvenile court judge and, based on the evaluating psychiatrist's report, had been remanded to a secure residential facility for treatment of their underlying emotional problems. Theoretically they would return to court for sentencing once their psychiatric problems had been addressed. In practice, they usually remained at the secure facility until their eighteenth birthday and were then either transferred to the adult correctional system or turned loose. This decision, Bernard explained, was based more on the presiding judge's attitude and mood than on the youth's psychiatric status.

Lately there had been fewer adjudicated children referred to Possum Ridge, and only a fraction of those youngsters were released when they reached voting age.

Bernard also pointed out that nearly every residential treatment center in the Northeast had named their facilities' units after trees.

Possum Ridge, having chosen an animal moniker for the entire school, was no exception. I found myself wondering why they had named this unit for a tree that had been virtually wiped out by disease.

As we entered the Elm Unit Bernard said hello to two large men who were leaving. "The guy on the right is Dave Porter. He's the one who discovered Kevin's body."

"No kidding. Do you think I could ask him a few questions?"

Bernard shrugged, then looked around to see if anyone was watching. "Hey, hold up a minute."

We caught up with the two men and Bernard introduced us, explaining that I was a private investigator who was helping Tommy's family find out what happened the night of Kevin's death. I appreciated his acknowledgment of my professional status, but wished he had been less specific in identifying me. People generally don't like to speak to investigators, public or private. Dave briefly extended his hand. His smile was forced and his grip a bit too firm, but I preferred his greeting to what I got from his companion. The other man, who Bernard called Jack, stood with his arms folded across his chest, looking as if I had accused his mother of having more than a casual interest in four-legged farm animals.

"I understand you were the first person to find Kevin," I said. "I'd be grateful if you could describe exactly what you saw that night."

Dave glanced at Jack who frowned. Jack was obviously a man of few words and many nasty expressions. "I don't know", Dave said. "I've told the police everything I know several times. Why don't you read their report?"

"I have, but there are still a few things I'm not clear on. I was hoping you might be able to fill in some of the details."

This time Dave looked at his watch. "I've got to run a group in five minutes. I don't have time to tell you the whole story but I'll try to answer a couple of quick questions."

Jack scowled and I jumped in before he could flash me the evil eye. "When you came into the room, where was Tommy?"

"He was sitting on the bed," Dave responded.

"It was a double room, right?" I said.

"That's right."

"Which bed?" I asked.

It took a second for my question to register. "Tommy was sitting on the bed on the left as you come into the room. He was near the head of the bed, right before the pillow."

"And Kevin?"

"He was lying in between the two beds with his head toward the back of the room." Dave glanced at his watch again. "Is that all? I really have to get to the unit. Besides I just remembered that Harrington told me I shouldn't speak to anyone without someone from administration present."

"Just one more question," I pleaded. "I'm sure Ms. Harrington won't object. She's the one who brought me over to speak with Bernard." This time Dave didn't seek counsel from the face of his watch. He merely shrugged, which I interpreted as permission to proceed. "In your statement you said that Tommy was holding the knife. Do you remember how he was holding it?"

Dave chewed on his finger as he tried to reconstruct the murder scene. "I'm not completely sure. I think he was holding it by the handle with his arm at his side. As I recall he was holding it like this." He pulled a ballpoint pen out of his pocket and gripped it in his fist. "The handle was here," he said, pointing to the clicker between his thumb and forefinger. "And the blade stuck out this way," he explained, touching the tip of the pen that protruded from the fleshy side of his hand.

"Which hand?" I asked.

"His right hand," Dave said tentatively. "Yeah, his right hand," he repeated with more confidence.

"You sure?" I asked.

"Yeah. I'm certain."

Bernard, who had been quietly observing our conversation, cleared his throat. I looked over at him and he raised his eyebrows but didn't say anything. Dave looked at his watch again and told me he had to go. I thanked him for his help and shook his hand, pulling mine away before he had a chance to pulverize it. Jack, remaining in character, grunted and tossed me a scornful look as he followed Dave.

When they were out of earshot I turned to Bernard and asked, "What do you think?"

"Dave's not too bright but he's a decent guy. He's always been straight with me. Of course, Harrington's been putting the heat on the staff to keep this as low profile as possible. The school's got enough problems without this. The last thing she wants is a full-blown scandal. Damage control is at the top of her agenda and I'm sure she's leaned on Dave to volunteer as little as possible."

"You think he might be holding back some details?"

"Hard to tell." Bernard began to fidget. "We better get you to Clover's office before Harrington sends out the hounds."

I couldn't tell if Bernard was really concerned or had just exceeded his quota of sedentary behavior, but decided not to push the issue. "Okay," I said. "Lead the way. Incidentally, what was that little eyebrow gesture you gave me when Dave was telling me about the knife?"

"No big deal. Just something he said seemed odd."

"And what might that be?" Bernard obviously enjoyed drawing out the suspense.

"Dave said he was holding the knife in his right hand."

"And?"

"Tommy's a southpaw. He eats with his left hand, writes with his left hand. The one time I saw him throw a ball, I'm pretty sure it was with his left hand."

"Hmm. That's interesting. Good observation, Bernard. You ought to give some thought to becoming a private investigator."

"You're kidding me."

"No, I'm serious. Having a good eye for detail is one of the most important requisites for the job."

"That's not what I mean," Bernard said, shaking his head. "Wasn't that what you were getting at with all those questions you were asking Dave? If Tommy had stabbed Kevin, the knife would have been in his left hand."

"No, actually I was focusing on the point of entry. Kevin was stabbed on the left side of the chest. The police report mentioned the knife penetrated at an angle, toward his left shoulder, which suggests the person who stabbed him used his left hand. The fact that Tommy had the knife in his right hand raises some doubts. Unfortunately, his southpaw status works against him in this instance."

"Oh shit," Bernard said disgustedly. "I thought I was helping Tommy."

"Don't lose hope yet. The burden of proof is on the prosecutor. He still has to explain why Tommy had the knife in his right hand. Granted it's not much, but every shred of doubt helps."

Doubt was definitely not in short supply, at least in my mind. How come I hadn't thought of finding out which hand Tommy used? My profound observation that the burden of proof rested on the D.A.'s shoulders might have reassured Bernard. But it didn't give me much solace. What if Bernard hadn't noticed that Tommy was holding the knife in his non-dominant hand. I would have felt more than a little foolish when the prosecutor pointed out in court that my theory about why Tommy couldn't have stabbed Kevin with his right hand, given the trajectory of the knife, actually added credence to their case against the left-handed defendant.

It crossed my mind that I might benefit from signing up for a refresher course from the Ablemann School.

When we reached Dr. Clover's office Bernard shook my hand and told me to call him if I had any questions. He seemed anxious to leave before I knocked on Clover's door, but knowing his hyperactive nature I didn't think much of it. I thanked him for the information on Tommy and told him I would probably follow up with him in the next few days. As he bounded down the hall I repeated my suggestion that he consider a career as a private investigator. I didn't offer to turn Tommy's case over to him, though at that moment I was tempted.

My knock on the door was greeted by a resonant voice inviting me to enter. I opened the door, stepped into the office, and did a double take. The person seated in the large leather chair in the corner of the room was the spitting image of Harold Prosic. Both doctors were exceptionally large in stature and wore their thick brown hair in the same slicked back fashion. The resemblance did not end with their physical features. Like Prosic, Dr. Clover also wore a dark gray pinstripe suit with a white shirt. I could not recall the precise pattern of Prosic's tie, but remembered that it was red, just like Clover's.

After Clover motioned me to sit in a matching chair I quickly discovered that the two mental health professionals were not identical in all ways. They differed in at least two respects.

The first distinction was their mental status. Unlike Prosic, who seemed to be engaged in a scintillating conversation with the ceiling, his look-alike was sharp and focused. From the moment I sat down Clover's eyes bore into me like a laser beam. Clover was direct without being hostile, intelligent and insightful but not distant and cold like some intellectuals I have known. In fact, Clover's empathy was so intense I immediately wanted to reveal my most intimate secrets. Within the first two minutes of our discussion I was ready to consult with the good doctor on what I should do about Ollie. Only my professional integrity and an intense fear of looking like a fool kept me from baring my soul.

The second difference between the two doctors, which took slightly longer to discover, should have been more obvious to me. Dr. Clover was a woman.

Her first statement let me know just how perceptive she was. "Surprised?"

"What do you mean?" I responded, hoping that I wasn't that transparent and wondering which surprise she was referring to.

"Gloria Harrington told me that you met with Dr. Prosic. You aren't the first person to notice the resemblance."

"Yes, I did notice some superficial similarity," I said, relieved that she had picked up on her resemblance to Prosic rather than her gender. "Your suit, for instance, is almost the same color as his."

She smiled. "Very good, Mr. Fenton. Given your line of work I'm certain your powers of observation are quite keen. How long did it take you to figure out that I am a woman?"

As the TV sitcom stars say, I didn't want to go there.

"As Ms. Harrington probably told you, I represent Tommy Hammond's parents. I'm trying to get a sense of what kind of kid he is and how he was doing at Possum Ridge. Of course my real purpose is to find out what happened the night Kevin Landry was killed and why Tommy was sitting in that boy's room with a knife in his hand. Any insight you can provide will be appreciated."

Clover's eyes locked into mine. I couldn't tell if she was deciding whether to trust me, playing head games with me, or simply composing a response. Whatever she was trying to do, it felt like she was reading my mind; which, if you haven't had the experience, is a strange sensation. Perhaps even stranger was that I was getting used to her apparent ability to know what was going on within my head and it didn't really bother me.

I wasn't yet ready to talk about Ollie, however.

"You've got a tough job," she said finally. "The evidence seems clear-cut, at least on the surface, and Tommy's illness limits his ability to advocate for himself. Part of me believes, or maybe wants to believe, that Tommy didn't do it. Unfortunately I can't produce any tangible evidence to support that belief." She picked up a thick folder from her desk and held it in her hands as if she were weighing the packet. "I guess that's what you're here for, to find some hard evidence, something that will help Tommy."

"That's right. I was hoping you could help me. As his doctor…" I glanced up at the diplomas on the wall. "As his psychiatrist, you probably know more about Tommy than anyone at the school. Is there anything about him that might give us a clue about what happened that night?"

Dr. Clover shifted in her seat. I sometimes wondered what it would feel like to be obese. Not just how people would respond to you or how you would feel when you walked into a room and adults began to whisper to each other while their children, who had not yet been socialized to mask their responses, giggled mercilessly. It was the concrete practical aspects of obesity that drew my attention: how a person of Dr. Clover's size navigated a narrow passageway or squeezed into a compact car or endured a transatlantic flight. Life is hard enough without these extra hassles.

"Just what kind of clue are you looking for?" she asked. "A telltale Rorschach response? A dark spot on his brain scan? Or maybe Tommy revealed a deep seated hostility toward Kevin in his play therapy session?"

"I . . . I'm not sure what kind of clue I'm looking for," I said, sinking down into my seat. "I just thought you might have picked up something that could help me understand what happened."

"I hate to disappoint you, but I don't have any clues for you. Clues are for board games and Hercule Poirot and for private investigators like yourself. Psychiatrists don't operate on the basis of clues. We use empirical data when we can put our hands on it and occasionally are fortunate to be blessed with a valid insight. Mostly we plod along, hoping to find some combination of psychotropic medication and psychological therapy that will give our patients some small relief from their personal demons. As for understanding what a child is capable of doing, past behavior is the best predictor of future actions. In Tommy's case, there is no shortage of explosive incidents in his record, even during his stay at Possum Ridge. But as far as I know, he never before attacked anyone with a knife. Does that mean he's incapable of stabbing another child? No, it's not beyond the realm of possibility. Not for Tommy, not for me and I suspect not even for you."

"So where does that leave us?" I chose to ignore her reference to my violent propensities. My reaction to Ollie and Lars had definitely tarnished my image of myself as a rational being.

Clover pushed herself up from the chair and walked to a small table on the other side of the room. She picked up a ceramic pot that was plugged into the wall receptacle. "Can I interest you in a cup of tea or hot chocolate?" Fearing that I might offend her, I asked for a cup of tea. She placed tea bags in two delicate porcelain cups and filled them with hot water. She handed me a cup and returned to her seat. She took a cup of tea and placed the cup on the end table next to her chair. Following her lead I raised the tea cup and drank. The hot liquid scalded my lip.

Dr. Clover smiled at me. I was certain she knew I had burned my mouth. "Where that leaves us, Mr. Fenton, is in a hard place. There are no facts to support your hypothesis that Tommy did not stab Kevin Landry. The police have a pile of circumstantial evidence supporting their hypothesis that Tommy killed Kevin. As far as I know they don't have another suspect. I doubt if they're even looking for one. And as you know, although the police use rigorous methods to gather evidence, their investigative activities are sometimes influenced by other forces: the pressure to close cases quickly, for instance."

My tongue was becoming numb and I was irritated by Clover's pedantic observations. The fact that her assessment was accurate didn't help my disposition. "It's easy for you to sit there and pontificate about the virtues of the scientific approach and the abuses it suffers in the hands of the working class. Unfortunately, it doesn't do anything for

121

Tommy Hammond. I was hoping you might suggest who I might speak with or where I should look to get more information. He is your patient, isn't he?"

Several large red blotches appeared on Clover's neck. "I can see where you might misunderstand what I am saying. I don't mean to be difficult. I know you're doing your best to help Tommy. It must be very frustrating for you. Nevertheless I can't manufacture useful information. Tommy is a loner. He didn't interact with the other kids and the staff were happy when he responded to their most basic instructions. I think I know Tommy better than anyone at Possum Ridge knows him and I don't have the vaguest idea what goes on inside his head."

Her words were not reassuring but her conciliatory gesture made me feel less irritable. I took another sip of tea. This time I didn't scald my mouth. "What about Bernard Washington? He seems to have a good feel for Tommy. He told me he's certain Tommy didn't kill Kevin."

"I hope I don't provoke your ire," Clover said with a faint smile, "but you've just made my point for me."

"What point is that?" I asked, uncertain whether I should allow my ire to be provoked.

"The unreliability of predicting behavior. To be more precise, the problem of assuming that a person's subjective view of another person's action actually has a factual basis."

"Huh?"

"I'm sorry," Clover said, shaking her head. "I guess I do have a pedantic streak, though I prefer to characterize it as a flair for provoking curiosity."

"I'm beginning to think that your real flair is provoking people's ire."

Clover peered at me. "You're not angry at me, are you?"

Disarmed again. "Not really. I just wish you'd make your point. It's been a long time between donuts and my stomach's beginning to growl."

"Okay, I'll get to the point. My point is that your informant is not totally objective. Bernard Washington is an excellent counselor. I can't think of anyone who relates as well as he does to the kids, especially those who are severely disturbed. But he tends to over-identify with them. He sees them as victims of the system. According to Bernard, if schools were less rigid, social service agencies more compassionate, and mental health professionals more willing to leave the security of their offices and get out into the community, most of these kids wouldn't be in residential treatment."

"Is he right?"

"There's some truth in what he says, but he extends this line of reason too far. He refuses to believe that any of these children are capable of initiating an aggressive act."

Her logic was plausible, but did not alter my positive opinion of Bernard. "To borrow a page from your lecture," I said, "where's the empirical data to support your assessment of Washington? What makes you think he has a biased viewpoint?"

As soon as I finished speaking, I knew I had been set up. Grinning like a Cheshire, Clover said, "My empirical data—and I am flattered that you would borrow my phrase—is that Bernard Washington spent most of his childhood right here, as a resident of Possum Ridge School."

CHAPTER TWELVE

It's better at home. Mommy and daddy are nice to me. They give me comics books. They give me ice cream. It's not nice here. I must be very bad. Why don't they let me go home?

Not wanting to prolong my embarrassment I quickly thanked Dr. Clover for her help, said I might contact her later, and headed for the parking lot. My confidence in Bernard had not been completely shattered, but Dr. Clover's zinger had certainly raised some serious questions.

I was still preoccupied with Clover's closing comment as I turned the key in the ignition and shifted into reverse. As soon as I began to back up I heard a thumping sound. I got out of the car to check the tires. The two on the driver's side were fine, but the rear tire on the passenger side was completely flat.

Remembering that I had forgotten to replace my spare the last time I had a flat tire, I kicked the wheel, muttered a few expletives and stormed off to find a telephone. As bad as yesterday had been with Lars and the toothless old man in the toilet stall, today was shaping up to be even worse. And it was barely noon.

The receptionist in the administration building was kind enough to let me use her phone. I was supposed to meet Ollie for lunch in less than ten minutes and was hoping to catch her before she left for the restaurant. Either my luck was turning or the gods were lulling me into a false sense of well-being before socking me with a mega dose of misfortune. As I dialed the number to Lars' studio I tried to ignore the little voice that was telling me Ollie had made up the story about him being gay and was at that moment jumping his Scandinavian bones on his king size waterbed.

To my relief Ollie picked up the phone on the second ring, sparing me the embarrassment of speaking with Lars.

After laughing at my latest round of misfortune Ollie said she would ask Lars if she could borrow his car and would ride out to rescue me as soon as possible. I asked if she had enough money to pick up an inexpensive replacement tire. She told me she didn't know if she could bring me another tire and suggested I look for a big wad of gum instead.

When I returned to my car the tire was still flat and the spare tire was still missing. As I puttered around in the trunk a nagging doubt began to form in the back of my mind. Dr. Clover had made a strong impression on me. While she bore an uncanny resemblance to Harold Prosic, the similarity ended there. She was clear and decisive while he came across as uncertain and vague. She tuned in to even the most subtle emotional cues while he appeared to be oblivious to everything but the scene on the ceiling of his office that only he could see.

In addition to having a barely controllable urge to pour my soul out to her, I was fascinated by the clarity of her mind. In spite of Dr. Clover's unfeminine appearance there was something about her that I could only describe as seductive. She had bombarded my senses with provocative insights, and led me down the cold, narrow path of logical positivism. I had struggled against her potent arguments, refusing to succumb to her scientific embrace. Just as I thought I had eluded her cynical grasp, she unleashed a powerful salvo of empirical evidence that brought me to my knees.

At the time Clover told me about Bernard Washington it made perfect sense that he could not be right about Tommy's innocence. Bernard was not an objective observer. He had been a resident of Possum Ridge so he could not possibly be considered a credible source.

Now, as I detached the jack from the trunk of the Honda, her argument did not seem as appealing. Looking back at our conversation I realized that Dr. Clover had not told me anything about Tommy other than a few general statements about his social behavior. Nor had she said anything substantive about herself. Applying Clover's own logic that one needed to consider the source, I wondered what personal bias or ulterior motive shaped Clover's response. Could I trust her? Was she being honest with me? Maybe she had invented the story about Bernard being a resident of

Possum Ridge just to deflect attention away from her own involvement in Kevin's murder.

My train of thought was interrupted by the sound of laughter. I turned to see the offensive line of the New York Giants coming toward me. At least they could have passed for a football team. There were five of them: four men—two white and two black—and a woman. They were roughhousing with each other as they approached me. One of the black men punched a white man on his shoulder. The second white man turned and jabbed at the woman's upper arm. She whirled around and socked him in the stomach. He doubled over and the others howled with laughter.

The black man who had thrown the punch noticed me standing by the car with a jack in my hand. "Hey, buddy, everything okay?"

"Other than having a flat tire, everything is fine."

"Can we give you a hand?"

"No thanks, I've got it under control," I lied.

The man who had been sucker-punched straightened up and looked at me. It was scowling Jack, the unhappy fellow who had given me the evil eye as we spoke with Dave, the counselor who had discovered Kevin's body. The sympathy I felt for him being punched in the stomach immediately disappeared. "That's the private investigator I was telling you about; the guy who's snooping around asking questions about Kevin Landry and Tommy Hammond."

The five of them closed in around me. Up close, they looked even larger. Although she was not as big as the four men, the woman was the most intimidating member of the gang. She was as wide as she was tall and looked as if she could bench press me without any difficulty. She had a square flat face with a bent nose that looked as if it had been the victim of a lucky punch. I didn't envy the person who had landed that blow. She stood directly in front of me bouncing on the balls of her feet, smacking her fist into her palm. She glared at me with eyes that dared me to return her stare.

I looked down at my feet.

"Why do you have to stick your nose into our business?" one of the men asked. I don't think he wanted an answer.

"Yeah," said the man who had initially offered to help me. "We have enough problems at the school without your stirring up trouble.

Harrington tells us the state might pull our license if the school gets any more bad publicity."

"I don't think they'd revoke your license because I'm asking a few questions," I said. "Besides..."

"You don't listen very good, do you?" the stocky woman said, stepping closer. She continued to pound her fist into her other hand. "We don't need nobody stirring up any trouble. We like our jobs and we don't intend to lose them because of some nosey investigator."

I was curious about what kind of job she had that she liked so much. Chief thumb screw turner? Dean of discipline?

Jack, who had been practicing his nastiest scowl, stepped forward and put his finger under my nose. "In case you have a problem understanding what we're saying, let me put this to you in plain English. We don't want you coming around asking dumb questions. We don't want you here at all, period. Is that clear?"

His words were clear, which was more than I could say for his breath. I hadn't smelled anything that rotten since I left an egg salad sandwich in my dormitory room during spring break. Maybe that was why Jack was always scowling.

The driver of a passing car honked but I ignored it. I was too nervous to take my eyes off the irate group surrounding me. Part of me wanted to tell them they ought to be ashamed of themselves for trying to thwart the efforts of the one person who was looking after Tommy Hammond's best interest. I rejected that inclination, however. The message was not likely to be well received. Besides, it was sort of self-righteous.

Another part of me was tempted to bolt through the wall of flesh and run like hell. The image of being gang-tackled by this angry mob dissuaded me from exercising this option.

As I was searching for a more rational part of me deep within the recesses of my psyche, I caught a glimpse of Ollie rolling a tire toward me. I debated whether to signal her to turn around and get help. Knowing Ollie, however, I was certain that my warning would backfire and make her more determined to handle the situation by herself.

"Hi Marty," she said cheerfully. "Find some friends to help you change your tire?" She was dressed in a turtleneck sweater, an oversized flannel shirt that must have been Lars' and a baggy pair of sweat pants. She looked tiny next to the Possum Ridge staff.

"Who is she?" Jack asked, looking at Ollie disdainfully.

"She must be a junior investigator," the large woman observed. She stopped her fist pounding, reached over and patted Ollie on the head. "Such a good girl, fetching your hero's tire while he looks for clues."

Ollie gave me a puzzled look. I shrugged. "Please don't do that," she told the husky woman in a calm voice.

"What's the matter?" the woman responded. "Afraid I might muss up your nice hair?" Again she extended her hand toward Ollie's head. This time Ollie stepped back beyond her reach.

"Grace," said the man who had first punched Jack in the arm, "I don't think the little lady appreciates your friendly gesture."

"Maybe she thinks you like her," Jack chimed in. "She probably thinks you have . . . shall we say, a romantic interest in her."

Their taunting had its desired effect. Grace's face turned red and her eyes narrowed. "Is that what you think?" Ollie shook her head. Other than the pulsating vein on the side of her neck, a warning sign that she was becoming angry, Ollie appeared to be completely at ease.

"I guess she doesn't think you're good enough for her, Grace," Jack said, adding fuel to the smoldering fire.

Grace stared at Ollie. She had resumed her fist-pounding posture. The tension was hard to miss.

"How about we go for lunch. We're going to be late if we don't move our sorry asses." The suggestion was made by one of the two men who hadn't previously spoken, a tall black man with a thick mustache.

"There you go, Floyd," the other black man said, "thinking about your stomach again. You can grab a sandwich if you want. I'm staying right here. I think this is going to be more satisfying than a turkey club."

Sensing that any effort to defuse the situation was futile, the tall black man shrugged and fell silent.

Grace glanced over her shoulder to see if anyone else was in the parking log. Seeing no one she turned back to Ollie and said, "I don't like your attitude."

"I don't have an attitude," Ollie responded. "I don't have a problem with you. I'm simply trying to tell you I would appreciate it if you didn't touch me."

128

I could feel the tension escalating, but felt helpless to do anything about it. Grace was determined to provoke Ollie or force her to yell Uncle, and her friends were happy to egg her on. I knew that Ollie would not back down and I didn't feel comfortable with the odds even though I knew Ollie could take care of herself.

"So you would appreciate me not touching you," Grace said, moving closer to Ollie. "Well I don't appreciate the way you're talking to me."

Three of the men moved behind Ollie, blocking the view from the school. Only Floyd didn't move. He looked almost as uncomfortable as I felt.

"Listen, I don't know what's going on," Ollie said. "All we want to do is change a tire and be on our way. If I've done something to offend you, I'm sorry. I certainly didn't mean any harm. Why don't we declare a truce. If you'll let us get to the car we'll be out of your way in a few minutes."

"That sounds okay with me," Grace said, turning sideways and gesturing for Ollie to pass. Ollie picked up the tire and took a step toward the car. With lightening speed Grace swirled and lunged at Ollie, pushing her forcefully with both hands. Ollie stumbled backwards, lost her grip on the tire, and fell to the ground.

"I'm sorry," Grace said bouncing on her feet like a prize fighter. "I have a bad sense of direction."

Ollie sat where she fell, looking up at Grace. Her face was as expressionless as it had been throughout the confrontation. Grace continued bouncing, waiting for the referee to count Ollie out. After a moment, Ollie dusted off her sweat pants and slowly rose to her feet.

Once again, Grace lunged at Ollie. This time Ollie was prepared. She ducked under Grace's outstretched arms and shot an elbow into the large woman's stomach, driving her backward. Grace staggered but did not fall.

Grace took several deep breaths as she glared at Ollie. She rubbed her hands together. "Okay, sister, you want to play. That's fine with me."

"That's enough, Grace," Floyd said, stepping forward.

The other black man held up his hand. "Don't be a killjoy, Floyd. They're just having fun." The two white men nodded. Floyd shook his head and stood back.

It took me a few seconds to locate the growling sound. Grace had

129

moved into a crouch, arms extended, head tucked in, and she was making a low guttural sound like a dog who's been backed into a corner. Ollie looked at her quizzically but did not move.

Without warning Grace sprung out of her crouch and raced toward Ollie. I thought Ollie would step aside and try to trip the larger woman. Instead she slid her right foot back and lowered herself into a crouch. Just as Grace was about to crash into her, Ollie straightened up and grabbed one of the charging woman's wrists. At the same time she stepped to the side and yanked Grace's arm back in the direction she had come from. The momentum spun both women around, though neither lost her footing.

After nearly a full rotation Grace planted her feet and swung her free arm down toward Ollie's head. Ollie removed one hand from Grace's wrist and grabbed her other hand. At the same time she hooked her foot behind Grace's ankle. Then Ollie jerked Grace's feet out from under her and yanked the large woman toward her.

Grace came crashing down on her knees.

Taking advantage of Grace's momentary disorientation, Ollie rearranged her grip, moving her palms flat against Grace's with their fingers intertwined. Since Grace was several inches taller than Ollie, their faces were close even in that position.

"We can call this off now," Ollie said, her breathing only slightly labored.

I didn't understand why Ollie said that. There was no way Grace was going to "call it off." Ollie must have known her diplomatic gesture would further provoke the volatile young woman.

"Up yours, asshole," Grace screamed. With brute strength, she pushed herself to her feet. For a second I thought her momentum would carry her forward and she would land on Ollie, squishing her like a bug. To my surprise Ollie held her ground. The two women stood face to face, hands locked together, each trying to bend the other's wrists back and down.

"Come on Grace, break her fucking arm."

"You got her now. Stomp that bitch into the ground."

The words of encouragement came from her cheering section. I wanted to say something supportive to Ollie, to help her overcome Grace's home court advantage, but the best I could do was mumble, "You're okay, Ollie." The whole situation seemed unreal.

The two women pushed against each other fiercely. Grace's face turned beet red. Ollie's complexion did not change but the protruding cords in her neck signaled the intensity of her exertion. They remained in stationary combat for what seemed like an eternity but in reality was probably no more than a couple of minutes. At first, Ollie seemed to have the edge, but Grace, with her extra height and weight soon pushed Ollie's arms back and gained the upper hand. They reversed positions several times with neither woman showing any signs of submitting. Just looking at them made me tired.

Suddenly Grace kicked out at Ollie's leg. Instead of stepping back, Ollie deftly slid to the outside of Grace's leg and at the same time pulled down on her hands. She released Grace's left hand, grabbed her right wrist with both hands and, with lightning speed, moved behind Grace and drove her arm up her back into a hammer lock. Ollie slipped her foot around Grace's legs and tripped her, forcing the large woman to her knees.

Ollie straddled Grace, pushing her arm further up her back. Other than uttering a grunt when she went down, Grace made no sound, though it was obvious from her facial expression that she was in considerable pain. Her companions did not look happy, either.

The pressure Ollie was applying to her twisted arm forced Grace's head down toward the ground. Ollie leaned down and whispered something into the fallen woman's ear. Grace did not respond. Ollie continued to whisper to her. I wished I knew what she was saying but dared not move closer, fearing I might provoke her three friends into taking retaliatory action. Floyd was clearly not in favor of their hostile behavior, but I didn't know if I could count on him to intervene if they decided to eat me for lunch. And if he did try to stop them he certainly couldn't count on me to be of assistance.

Ollie continued to apply pressure to the large woman's arm. Just before her head touched the ground, Grace nodded slightly. Ollie released her arm but did not move until she was sure Grace was not going to attack her again. Judging from Grace's quivering lips and the way she held her injured arm, the probability of her taking on Ollie at that moment was remote.

Ollie stepped away from Grace and looked at the three cheerleaders.

They looked down at the ground. "Aren't you going to help her?" Ollie asked. They moved clumsily toward Grace, but Floyd had already come to her side. He spoke to her softly.

"Does it hurt a lot?" He said gently as he knelt beside her.

She nodded.

"See if you can move it," he said. She moved it gingerly. "That's good. At least it's not broken. We better get you to the infirmary, though. Looks like you have at least a bad sprain."

"You're not going to tell them what happened." There was fear in Grace's voice. "If Harrington finds out I've been in a fight she'll fire me."

I made a mental note that it was Gloria Harrington and not Harold Prosic or any of the other supervisors who caused Grace to be frightened.

"Don't worry," Floyd said, "I won't tell her what happened. I sure am curious to hear your version of what happened. This is not your typical on-the-job injury."

Grace ignored his remark and turned to Ollie. "How about you? You going to report me?"

Ollie glanced at me and shrugged. "This is your business, Marty. I might have to fight your fight for you occasionally but I'm sure as hell not going to take responsibility for how you do your job."

That hurt.

"Let's put it this way," I said. "I have no need to get you in trouble as long as you don't interfere with my investigation. Any more threatening or getting in my way and I not only tell Ms. Harrington, I also talk to the assistant district attorney and the judge about how you are compromising my work as an officer of the court."

The last admonition was a bit of a stretch but we, or at least Ollie, was on a bit of a roll.

Grace nodded and muttered something that sounded like okay. I turned to the three men. They glared at me and didn't say anything. I interpreted their silence as an affirmative response, though my confidence in them being men of their word was not high.

As I watched Grace walk slowly back to the school with the four men, two tangential questions formed in my mind. What would happen to Floyd's status within this small circle of friends? My guess was that they would not think kindly of his unwillingness to join their assault on me.

My second question came more from my own growling stomach than from an innate sense of intellectual curiosity. How pissed would the three tough guys be when they realized they had blown their lunch hour watching their colleague being soundly thrashed by a woman half her size?

The sound of Ollie's voice brought me back to the source of my initial dilemma. "If you think I'm going to change your tire for you, too, you're sadly mistaken," she said caustically. I knew that remark about her changing the flat tire only scratched the surface of her frustration with me. Knowing this, I hesitated before telling her that neither of us was going to be changing the flat tire at that moment.

"We have a slight problem," I said, pointing to the tire. She looked at the tire trying to figure out what I meant. "Do you notice anything . . . unusual?"

"Stop screwing around, Marty. I'm in no mood for one of your puzzles, I'm tired and I just . . . " Her squint eyed glare let me know the light bulb in her head had just gone on. "Oh shit," she shouted. "Why didn't you tell me you needed the tire mounted on a rim?"

I wanted to say I had assumed she would know we needed a tire that was already mounted, but was afraid that would make her even angrier. Besides, that wasn't what happened. The truth was less flattering to me. Between my frustration from finding that the tire was flat and my fear that Lars might answer the phone, I had forgotten that there was no way to install a rimless tire in the middle of a parking lot. "I'm sorry," I said. "It slipped my mind. Do you think we could stop at a service station?"

Ollie shook her head. "On one condition. You have to promise me you will invest some of the fee from this case into a Triple-A membership. None of this would have happened if you had renewed your membership."

I had enough sense not to argue with her.

The owner of the service station also happened to have a used auto parts lot which happened to have a rim that fit my Honda. It took fifteen minutes to locate the rim, ten minutes to mount the tire on the rim, and less than ten seconds to swipe my Visa card across the scanner. By the time I had driven back to Possum Ridge and changed tires we were both famished. I followed Ollie back to Northampton and we stopped at the first place we came to, a quiet Chinese restaurant on Pleasant Street.

After wolfing down a delicious dish of chicken and broccoli Ollie said she was going to walk to Lars' studio. To my surprise her announcement didn't bother me.

We agreed to meet for dinner. Ollie suggested we go to Spoleto's. Given the rave reviews she had given I said yes, told her goodbye and went off to look for a telephone.

Faith Pasternak answered on the second ring. She sounded pleased to hear from me and asked if I could come right over. Since the pay phone I was calling from was only three blocks from her office that did not pose a problem.

Faith greeted me with a firm handshake. I wanted to lean down and give her a hug, but wasn't sure how she would receive this gesture. I decided to wait until I knew her better.

"I've had a busy day," she said, wheeling herself over to her work station. "How about you?"

"Me too. I've had some interesting encounters."

"Good. I want to hear about them. But first let me fill you in on what I found. Okay?"

"Sure, fire away."

She picked up a folder from the desk and pointed toward a chair. She opened the folder and began to thumb through the pages. "This is a copy of the police report and the county attorney's indictment report. They're as interesting for what they don't contain as for what they do. For starters, the police didn't bother to look for fingerprints at the crime scene. They didn't even check Kevin's clothing. After they tested to see if all of the blood on his shirt was Kevin's—which it was—his clothing mysteriously disappeared. The medical examiner remembers running the test but can't recall seeing them after the autopsy. Her assistant thinks they may have accidentally been placed in the discard bin."

"Pretty sloppy work. What did they find at the autopsy?"

"Cause of death was a sharp instrument penetrating through the lung and cutting the aorta. Nothing else remarkable. No bruises or other injuries. Several healed fractures: wrist, ankle, even collarbone . . . "

"Abuse?"

"Looks like it. Alcoholic father, ineffectual mother. Kevin was removed from his home by DSS two years ago. He's been in five foster home placements since then."

"Anything else?"

"Isn't that enough?"

"No," I said, realizing she had misunderstood me. "I'm talking about the autopsy."

"Oh. No, that's about it. No alcohol or other substances. Just the remains of an unappetizing Possum Ridge dinner."

"How about prescription drugs? Was Kevin on medication?"

"Good question. The report doesn't mention the presence of medication. Why don't you ask next time you talk to his psychiatrist?"

"Okay. What else doesn't the report address?"

"The police didn't bother to run any tests on Tommy. He had the knife in his hand; there was blood on the knife. Case closed. No fingerprint analysis of the weapon, no blood test on Tommy. Nothing. The Pioneer Valley doesn't have the swiftest law enforcement team in the country, but I've never seen anything as sloppy as this."

"Anything we can do about it?"

Faith shrugged. "Not much. It's too late to run any tests on Tommy. If there was anything in his blood it's gone by now. Darrow agreed to order a psychiatric exam for Tommy. I expect to hear the results any minute."

"Not much to go on. I was hoping you might uncover something."

"Me too," she sighed. "How about you? You have better luck?"

I recounted my meeting with Prosic and Harrington as well as my conversations with Bernard Washington and Dr. Clover. I omitted the encounter with Grace and her cronies. We made a list of next steps and divided the assignments between us. Faith told me she would call me at the motel if she received the results of the psychiatric exam. Otherwise we planned to meet for lunch the next day to brief each other.

Hopefully I wouldn't have another flat tire.

As I got up to leave, Faith slapped her forehead. "I almost forgot. I did pick up one interesting piece of information."

"What's that?"

"It might just be a coincidence, but I think it's worth pursuing."

She was really drawing out the suspense. "What might be a coincidence?" I asked, playing along.

"Where Kevin lived. He's the only other kid at Possum Ridge from Syracuse."

CHAPTER THIRTEEN

I put all my things on the shelf. I put them the way they're supposed to be. First the green truck, then the red car and the blue car. Then the motorcycle and the bus. Just how they're supposed to be. Then the mean people come and take it all down. That made me mad. Then they all hold me down. Not fair. I'm not hurting anybody. They should leave my things alone.

By the time I got back to the motel I was ready for a nap. The mattress wasn't any less lumpy than it had been the previous night but I was becoming accustomed to the room's eclectic charm.

I especially liked the art work. Ollie would appreciate the effect created by placing Picasso and Norman Rockwell side by side.

Before dropping off I made a mental note to ask the desk clerk if they honored frequent guest points.

I was awakened by the shrill ring of the antique rotary telephone.

"Hel . . . hello," I said groggily.

"Mr. Fenton, I'm glad I caught you. This is Gloria Harrington from Possum Ridge. I hope I'm not disturbing you."

"No, not at all. I was just resting."

"I can certainly understand that. You've had a busy day."

Did she know about the incident with Ollie and Grace? If so, her information couldn't have come from the fearsome five. They weren't about to let anyone know that Grace had been subdued by someone half her size. I had heard that institutional grapevines were awesome but hadn't actually seen one in action.

On the other hand, she might not know about the episode in the parking lot. Her remark about me having reason to be tired may have simply been a conversational ploy to gain my trust. By sympathizing with my hectic schedule she hoped I would see her as an ally, someone I could confide in.

Did graduate training in psychology instill paranoia or were suspicious people drawn to the study of behavior?

"What can I do for you, Ms. Harrington?" I asked, noticing that the Picasso print was hung upside down.

"I'm sorry I didn't get a chance to speak with you after your visit. I wanted to find out what you discovered. I . . . I also had something I wanted to share with you."

"Share away," I said, more sarcastically than I had intended.

"I was hoping to have a chance to speak with you privately," she said. "I was wondering if you might be free for lunch tomorrow. Or, if you're an early riser, there's a little place up the road that makes great French toast."

I suppressed my anger to tell her I was never free; it's hard to do pro bono work when your standard fee barely exceeds minimum wage. Instead I graciously agreed to meet her for lunch and made a mental note to change the time of my meeting with Faith.

I splashed water on my face and put on a clean shirt. I was on my way to the door when I remembered I hadn't called the Hammonds. Larry Hammond picked up the phone on the third ring, sounding even wearier than the last time we spoke. I brought him up to date on what little I had learned. He sounded so despondent I was tempted to tell him I had a few leads, but my conscience prevailed. Technically I had a few lines of inquiry I was pursuing, lunch with Gloria Harrington being one. But to call these legitimate leads would be stretching the truth.

Hammond asked how Tommy was doing. It was a difficult question to answer since I had not seen Tommy before and had a hard time picturing what normal was for him. I gave him a brief description of what I had observed.

I did not mention Tommy's comment that his parents didn't care for him.

After a brief consultation with his wife, Hammond told me they were coming to Northampton the next day. I asked if he wanted me to find a place for them to stay. He said that wouldn't be necessary. They had stayed in a nice place near Possum Ridge the last time they visited Tommy and he was sure they could get a room there. From his description I felt confident we wouldn't be staying at the same motel.

They planned to arrive in the late afternoon. I gave him my telephone number and asked him to call once they were settled. I promised to contact Faith Pasternak to arrange a meeting. Hammond thanked me and hung up. I could have been mistaken, but he sounded like he was on the verge of crying.

It was only after I was in my car driving to meet Ollie for dinner at Spoleto that the question emerged from the inner recesses of my brain: How did Gloria Harrington know where I was staying?

It didn't take long to figure out the origin of the restaurant's name. Posters of the annual Spoleto musical festival in South Carolina lined the walls. The mosaic tile mural on the bar and the colorful nautical mobiles hanging from the ceiling added to the festive ambiance of the dining room.

Even though it was not yet six o'clock, the restaurant was nearly full. I spotted Ollie and Lars at a table at the back of the restaurant. Taking a deep breath, I pulled back my shoulders and strode toward them. They both stood as I approached the table. Ollie kissed me on the cheek and Lars shook my hand. He had a huge hand and a firm grip. Mercifully he didn't squeeze too hard. I had the feeling he could have crushed my knuckles without much effort.

I sat next to Ollie, across from Lars. I noticed there was a fourth place setting.

"I hope you don't mind," Ollie said, "I invited Lars' nephew to join us for dinner. I was telling Lars about our visit to Possum Ridge and he told me his nephew works there. Isn't that weird? Makes you believe in the six degrees of separation theory, doesn't it?"

I shrugged.

Ollie wrinkled her brow. "Maybe he can give you some help," she said. "From what I saw the people at that school don't seem eager to tell you anything. Lars' nephew might know something that would be useful. Lars called him and he agreed to come. Don't worry, he didn't tell him that you were looking into the boy's murder. We didn't want to compromise your investigation. He only knows that I'm a former student of his uncle and you're . . . "

"Okay, Ollie," I said, not waiting to hear how she might describe me. "I appreciate you trying to help," I said to Ollie. "And thanks, Lars."

"No problem," Lars replied. "How about something to drink while we wait for my nephew?"

Ollie ordered a glass of white wine, Lars asked for a glass of Chianti, and I had a bottle of Sam Adams. We exchanged small talk for a few minutes. Lars asked what my thesis was about. I asked what he thought about Henry Moore, whom I had heard Ollie mention on several occasions. Ollie was smiling at my question and was about to speak when something behind me caught her attention. Her eyes widened and her jaw dropped.

As I turned to see what she was staring at, Lars rose and said, "Hi, I'm glad you could join us."

Standing next to the table was a tall, handsome young man with a mustache. There were two things about the young man that immediately caught my attention. The first was the color of his skin. I had expected Lars' nephew to be blonde, blue eyed with the ruddy complexion of someone who spends considerable time on the ski slope. Instead his nephew had dark hair, brown eyes, and skin that was nearly as dark as the wrought iron wine rack across from our table.

I suppose I should have been chagrined by having my stereotypical thinking exposed. Interracial marriage was not that uncommon, especially in a college community. But any embarrassment I might have experienced as a result of this affront to my self-image as an open minded individual was suppressed by the second surprise.

Lars' nephew was one of the men who had confronted Ollie and me in the Possum Ridge parking lot earlier that day.

Lars embraced his nephew. "Floyd, I want you to meet one of the best students I've ever had. This is Ollie Tolliver and her friend, Marty."

"We've already met," Floyd said, looking uncomfortable. "And if Ms. Tolliver can chisel wood as well as she can twist arms she must be one helluva sculptor."

"What do you mean, Floyd?" Lars said, looking puzzled.

Floyd looked at Ollie. "You didn't tell him?"

Ollie shook her head.

"Will someone please tell me what's going on?" Lars pleaded.

Neither Ollie nor Floyd seemed eager to enlighten Lars. So I spoke up. "When we were at Possum Ridge this morning a group of staff decided they didn't like me snooping around their school. They confronted me in the parking lot. One of the staff—the only woman in the group—decided to impress her colleagues. She got in Ollie's face, tried to provoke her. Ollie tried to walk away but the woman wouldn't give up. She kept getting nastier until Ollie couldn't ignore her."

"And you saw this, Floyd?" Lars asked.

"Uh . . . I . . . I was there."

"And you didn't do anything." Lars was glowering at his nephew.

"To tell you the truth, Ollie didn't need any help," Floyd said. "Grace is a pretty tough character but Ollie handled her like a piece of putty."

Remembering that Floyd had tried to defuse the situation I tried to come to his defense. "Floyd wasn't one of the instigators. In fact, he tried to get the others to back off."

Lars wasn't impressed. "I'm surprised at you, Floyd. You know too well what can happen in a situation like that. You should have stopped it." Lars turned to Ollie. "Did you get hurt?"

Ollie had been slouched in her chair looking down at the table as Lars grilled his nephew. Now she blushed. I wasn't surprised that she hadn't told Lars about the incident at Possum Ridge. She didn't like to draw attention to herself, and became uncomfortable when anyone focused on her physical prowess. This didn't didn't make sense to me, but there was lot about Ollie that puzzled me.

"I'm fine, Lars," Ollie said quietly. "And Marty's right. Floyd tried to call off the others. I don't think he could have done anything else. Now can we order some food? I'm famished."

Lars signaled our server, a vivacious young woman with shoulder-length blonde hair who I guessed to be a student at Smith. When she first approached the table she had referred to him as Professor Olafson. Now, as she recited the specials for the day, Ollie, Floyd, and I might as well not have been there. She spoke directly to Lars and her eyes revealed that her interest went beyond attentive customer service.

There have been a lot of changes in higher education, but apparently students still had crushes on their professors. I wondered whether our server knew Lars was gay. Or if he really *was* gay.

We ordered appetizers and entrees and made small talk while we waited for the food. Lars told us that Floyd had graduated from the University of Massachusetts where he had been a wide receiver on the football team. At most universities this would have made him a campus celebrity. But at U-Mass basketball was king and football was a distant relative of the royal family. He had majored in sociology and minored in art. To Lars' chagrin, Floyd, who according to his uncle was a talented painter, had taken a job as a counselor at Possum Ridge rather than accepting a scholarship to study at a southern university whose fine art program had an excellent reputation.

In his defense, Floyd said he needed a break from school and might reapply for graduate school in a couple of years. He found his work with kids rewarding, though sometimes frustrating, and expressed doubt about whether he could make a living as an artist.

Just as Lars was about to challenge Floyd's view of his limited career potential in the arts, our appetizers arrived. At Lars' suggestion we had ordered baked stuffed artichokes with melted butter.

We ate silently for a few minutes, concentrating on the laborious but rewarding task of peeling, dipping, and sucking on the artichoke leaves, whose scant yield was tasty, but served primarily as a prelude to the meatier artichoke bottom and heart.

"Do you know why I was at Possum Ridge?" I asked Floyd, wiping my messy hands with a napkin.

"Sort of," Floyd replied. "As I understand it you're looking into Kevin Landry's death."

"That's basically right. Tommy Hammond's parents hired me. They're worried about their son and feeling helpless. They want to know what happened. They don't think Tommy would kill another child, but if he did, they're convinced there must have been a good reason. The police and the assistant district attorney aren't even pretending to go through the motions. They've got an easy suspect. Tommy was in the room with Kevin. He had a bloody knife in his hand. And given his emotional condition, he isn't going to say anything that might cause anyone to question his guilt. As far as the district attorney's office is concerned this is a no-brainer. Their only question is how to counter the defense attorney's argument that Tommy can't be held responsible for his actions because of his emotional state."

"Any chance they'll try him as an adult?" Lars asked.

"I don't know," I replied. "Massachusetts is a pretty liberal state but most states are treating juveniles charged with murder as if they're adults."

"Have you found anything yet?" Lars asked.

"Not really. Nothing solid enough to help Tommy."

"Do you know anything about this?" Lars asked Floyd.

"Nothing more than I read in the paper, Uncle Lars."

"I was hoping you might tell me something about the staff at Possum Ridge," I said. "I didn't expect them to greet me with open arms, but I received a pretty hostile reception, especially from your buddies. I also received a lot of conflicting opinions and I wasn't too impressed with the administrator. Frankly, I couldn't really tell who was in charge if, in fact, anyone is actually running the place."

At that moment our server arrived carrying a large tray on her shoulder. I couldn't help being impressed by her serving skills. Not only did she remember who ordered each dish. She also managed to unload the tray and place each dish properly without once taking her eyes off Lars.

The entrees were just as good as the appetizers. We ate silently for a few minutes, enjoying our meal. I was beginning to wonder if Floyd was trying to ignore my request when he put down his knife and fork, and wiped his mouth with a napkin. "The folks at Possum Ridge are mostly pretty decent."

"Mostly?" I asked, borrowing another trick from the instruction manual of my private investigator correspondence course.

Floyd squirmed in his seat. "I'm not saying they're perfect, but it's a tough job working with these kids. They know how to push your buttons. A lot of the staff are stressed out."

I was willing to let Floyd wind down for awhile but his uncle wasn't. "If you know anything that might help that poor boy they have locked up, now is the time to tell Mr. Fenton," Lars said, putting his hand on his nephew's shoulder.

Damn. I was beginning to like Lars in spite of myself.

Floyd sighed before he spoke. "You're partially right about the administration. It's difficult to know who's running the center if you go strictly by job titles. You probably noticed that Dr. Prosic isn't all there." Floyd pointed to his head. "But there definitely is someone in charge."

"Gloria Harrington?" I guessed.

Floyd nodded. "She's the assistant director," he explained to Lars and Ollie. "Worked her way up from being an intake worker. She seems to know what she's doing. I guess the school would be in bigger trouble than it is if it weren't for her. There's something about her though. I don't trust her."

I filed his comment about the school being in trouble in my memory bank. "Has she given you any reason not to trust her?"

Floyd started to shake his head but stopped midway. "There was this one incident last fall. It might not have meant anything but it struck me as odd at the time. We were having an all-school assembly. We have three or four a year. We gather all the kids in the auditorium, usually in the early afternoon. Evening staff are required to come in a couple of hours early to help manage the kids. They don't usually mind. They pick up a little overtime.

"The administration tells the kids about changes they are planning to make. Building renovations, revising the behavior modification point system, that kind of thing. Then they give everyone a little pep talk. 'This is the best group of kids and staff Possum Ridge has ever had. We're going to have a great year!' Something like that. Then they put on a show for the kids. Most of the time they bring in an outside group, a theater group or a choir.

"The incident I remember took place after the show. The kids had just seen a performance by a local church drama group. It was some kind of morality play about kids making the right choices. Drugs, sex, cheating in school; a little hokey, but pretty well done. Even had some upbeat music; Christian rock, I guess. The kids were pumped up. I'm not sure it was the message that got to them. More likely it was the music and the good-looking lead actors, male and female.

"Harrington was trying to get the kids to settle down and wasn't having much luck. Dr. Clover, one of the shrinks, vaulted onto the stage and began talking to the kids about the play. Doc told them the play had

143

an important message for them. They had to learn to make their own choices. If they made bad choices that were going to get in trouble and would spend a long time in places like Possum Ridge—or worse. Unless they learned to make decisions that were in their best interest there wasn't much hope for them."

At that moment our server returned to ask if we were enjoying out dinners. As she refilled our water glasses she kept her eyes on Lars, who appeared to be unaware of her interest in him. Lars asked how her studies were going. The young woman, surprised by his attention to her, became unsettled. As she turned to compose a coherent response, her hand began to shake. Unfortunately she was, at that instant, pouring water into my glass. The water missed the glass, splashed on to the table, and flowed onto my lap. The server apologized profusely and hurried off to find some napkins.

Ollie, who had not been oblivious to the server's interest in Lars, leaned over and whispered in his ear. Lars' face turned red. Noticing that our server was returning, he excused himself and hurried off to the men's room.

It was becoming more difficult not to like Lars.

As I blotted my trousers, Floyd continued his story about the school assembly. "The kids were actually responding to Clover's talk. They had quieted down and seemed to be thinking. Harrington wasn't too pleased though. She stood off to the side, arms folded across her chest, looking like she was constipated."

"That doesn't make sense," Ollie said. "You'd think she would be happy that the kids had settled down, especially if they were paying attention to Dr. Clover's message."

"You'd think so," Floyd said. "But she wasn't. And she was even less pleased with what happened next. Doc Clover told the kids they should pay attention to the play's message about making good choices but then went on to say that the play's other message, that they should follow Jesus and the New Testament, might not be suitable for all of them. Some of the kids are Jewish, a few are Muslim, and I wouldn't be surprised if there were a couple who don't believe in any religion. Doc told the kids it didn't matter what religion or set of beliefs they based their choices on as long as they had a decent set of values that allowed them to act in their own best interest without hurting others."

"Sounds reasonable," I said.

"Harrington didn't think so," Floyd said. "She practically knocked Doc Clover over getting to the microphone. She told the kids that everything in the play was important, that they shouldn't pay attention to some parts and ignore others. Then she dismissed the kids. She said something to Clover and I don't think she was thanking Doc for enlightening the kids. She looked pretty angry. Before Doc could respond she hurried over to apologize to the leader of the drama group who was still sitting at the back of the stage."

"You think she was embarrassed?" Ollie asked. "I can see Clover's point, trying to be sensitive to the diversity of the students. But I can also understand how she would worry that her guests might take the doctor's remarks out of context and see them as being critical of their religion."

Floyd shook his head. "That's a generous interpretation, Ms. Tolliver. I think Harrington was more upset that Doc had upstaged her. As I said before, she pretty much runs the place. For Clover to step in when she was trying to settle them down didn't please her. The fact that they listened to Doc when they hadn't to her made her even angrier."

"Pretty insecure woman," Ollie observed.

"You bet," Floyd said. "She has a wicked temper and a memory that doesn't quit. You don't want to get on her bad side. She holds a grudge forever."

"Beside the fact that she reamed out Clover, was there anything else about the incident that caused you to be suspicious of Gloria Harrington?" I asked.

"Oh yeah," Floyd said. "Definitely. If it had ended there I wouldn't have thought much of what happened. Conflict between staff is not uncommon, even among administrators. Later that afternoon I stopped by the personnel office to check on my leave time. On my way I passed Harrington's office. I couldn't help overhearing what was going on inside. She was screaming at someone, saying their behavior was outrageous and unacceptable. The other person was speaking softly, maybe trying to calm her down. I couldn't tell who it was, but I'm pretty sure it wasn't one of the kids."

"You think it was Clover?" Ollie asked.

"I'm pretty sure," Floyd said.

"How sure?" I said.

"Let me put it this way. The assembly was held on Friday. I worked that weekend and was off Monday and Tuesday. When I came in Wednesday Dr. Clover's office was cleared out. I haven't seen him since."

At first I missed the significance of what Floyd had just said. I was too focused on his last words. "You said 'him.'"

CHAPTER FOURTEEN

Sometimes when the kids play ball the staff asks me to play. The other kids don't want me to play because I'm no good. Bernard tells them to be quiet and says I should try. I don't really want to play but I like Bernard. Then the kids make fun of me.

"That's right," Floyd said, sliding his chair in to make room for his uncle.

"I know Dr. Clover has a masculine appearance," I said, "but she told me she's a woman and I don't have any reason to doubt her."

Floyd looked puzzled for a few seconds. Then he broke into a broad grin. "Oh, you must have talked to the *other* Dr. Clover, the psychiatrist."

Ollie was having trouble following what both of us were saying. "There are two Dr. Clovers?"

Floyd was enjoying himself now. "Yeah, one more and we can name a plant after them. We could call it a three-leaf clover."

Lars frowned at his nephew, but couldn't conceal his grin. "How about giving us a more intelligent response."

Floyd shrugged. "Sure. Both Dr. Clovers have worked at Possum Ridge for years. She's the psychiatrist for mid- and late adolescents. He was the psychologist for the latency and early adolescent units. Mr. Fenton, you're the only one here who will appreciate this, since you met Dr. Clover, the woman. Physically they're the most unmatched couple I've seen in a long time. She's an extremely large woman and he's a wisp of a man, not much taller than five feet and probably less than a hundred pounds soaking wet. She moves like a snail; he's a hummingbird, never staying in one spot more than a few seconds."

147

At least I had solved one mystery: how Dr. Clover had managed to vault onto the stage. The Dr. Clover I met would have had difficulty stepping onto a scale.

"They look like an odd couple," Floyd said, "but they're both pretty neat people. When the kids first meet Mrs. Dr. Clover they're a little put off, but once they get to know her they can't wait for their sessions with her. Which really surprised me since her primary function is to manage the kids' medication and you know how much adolescents like to take meds. And then there's her style. You talked to her, Mr. Fenton, so you know what I mean. She's kind of formal, even cold. She thinks of herself as a scientist. Probably uses the words 'objective' and 'empirical' in every other sentence. Am I right?"

I nodded, remembering her scientific orientation, but also recalling how perceptive she was. It was almost as if she could read my mind. Ordinarily that would frighten adolescents, but in her case I could see how they might be drawn to her.

"Mr. Dr. Clover," Floyd continued, "is as different from his wife in personality as he is in physical appearance. He's kind of loosey-goosey, always kidding around with the residents. He participated in a lot of the activities with the kids. Had a pretty good arm in the outfield for a small man."

Floyd's description of the Clovers was interesting but I felt he was dragging it out deliberately. "What happened after Dr. Clover didn't return to school?" I asked. "What did his wife do?"

"Not much," Floyd said. "Granted she isn't one to show her feelings, but I didn't notice anything different about her." He paused for a few seconds. When he resumed, his voice was more animated. "There was one thing. Yeah, I almost forgot. Every Tuesday the professional staff holds a special clinical review meeting. They used to call it a case conference but one of the shrinks objected, said the kids weren't cases, they were people. They pick one child who has not responded well to the therapeutic program. The primary therapist usually gives a brief summary of the kid: where he or she came from, the problem that brought them to Possum Ridge, what's happened since they came here. Then all of the clinical staff sit around and talk about what's going on with the kid and what we might do to get him or her on track." Floyd stopped and looked around the table.

"I'm sorry. I'm talking too much. I'm kind of slow to get started, but once I begin I tend to get caught up in the details."

"What's wrong with details?" Lars asked. "I don't know a single artist with any talent who doesn't agonize over the details of his work."

"As long as the details are relevant," I said, immediately regretting that I had allowed myself to express my impatience.

Ollie gave me a scalding look. "Go on, Floyd, you're doing just fine."

"I'll try to speed it up," Floyd said self-consciously. "Dr. Clover—the psychiatrist—almost always runs these sessions. There are usually nine or ten professional staff and a few counselors. Most of the meetings are dull but sometimes the discussions are lively and occasionally they come up with good ideas for changing the kid's program."

"Does each child have a unique program?" Ollie asked. Her question was directed at Floyd but her half-smile was definitely for my benefit.

"Not really," Floyd replied. "There's a general milieu program which gives kids positive and negative consequences for their behavior. We use a point system. Kids earn points for appropriate behavior and are given bonus points for exceptional accomplishments like going out of their way to help another kid. Staff keep track of the points. If you earn a certain amount of points you can move to a higher program level which gives you more privileges like staying up later or going on special outings. Kids can also use their points to buy candy and toys at the school store."

"Is that what they call a token economy?" Lars asked. "I saw something recently on 20/20 or one of those other TV news magazines."

"Sort of," Floyd said. "Our program isn't very sophisticated. Probably could use some help from Alan Greenspan or some other high-powered economist. At one time we had a good point system but it's fallen off in the last couple of years, just like the rest of the program. Each kid is supposed to have individual target behaviors: using words to express anger, not setting up other kids, that sort of thing. Unfortunately, it's difficult to manage fifteen separate behavior modification programs on a unit. So unless there's a knowledgeable person in charge of the program, someone who constantly monitors what's happening, staff tend to focus all of their attention on milieu management. They do what it takes to make sure the unit is safe and running smoothly. Kids' individual goals get overlooked."

"You said the program used to be better," I said. "What's different now?"

"Lots of things," Floyd said sadly. "The most obvious difference is staffing. The school has serious budget problems and has reduced staffing by about twenty percent in the last couple of years—professionals as well as direct care and support staff. The first thing that drops off when staff is cut is the quality of attention each kid receives. In addition to not having enough coverage, staff are demoralized and don't have the resources or energy to do more than keep the kids in line."

"It must be discouraging," Ollie said.

"It is," Floyd agreed. "I used to enjoy doing my shift each day. I got a lot of satisfaction working with the kids. Now it seems like a struggle. The administration is constantly hassling us to be more efficient, the clinicians spend a lot of their time bickering with each other and most of the direct-care staff would leave if they could find other jobs."

Maybe Floyd's digression was not a waste of time. It sounded as if there were a lot of disgruntled employees at Possum Ridge. Could one of them have been frustrated enough to kill a child?

"I'm sure you don't want to hear about my job dissatisfaction," Floyd said." I'll try to stay on target. I happened to be at the clinical review meeting I was telling you about. There weren't many clinicians at the meeting, only four or five. But Gloria Harrington was there, which was unusual because she didn't usually come to the review sessions."

"Was Dr. Prosic there?" I asked.

"No, he never comes to the clinical meetings. In fact, I rarely see him outside of the admin building these days."

"That's strange," Ollie said. "You would think he'd want to see what's going on at the school."

Floyd shrugged. "They were talking about this kid who was having trouble adjusting to the school." He paused. "I'm a little uncomfortable talking about this. I don't want to violate confidentiality. The kids have few enough rights as it is. The least we can do is protect their privacy. The only way I can talk about this is if I don't mention names. Okay?"

We nodded.

"This kid was getting picked on by the other residents. Not just picked on. He was beat up on a regular basis. Nobody could figure out what was happening. Usually kids get picked on because they provoke the other kids: teasing, provoking, setting up..."

"You used that term a few times," Ollie said, "What does it mean to set up someone?"

Floyd scratched his head. "Jeez, How can I explain? It's like when someone tries to get two other people to fight with each other. A tells B that C is saying bad things about him. Then A goes to C and says that B is bragging that he can beat up C with one arm tied behind his back. Some of our kids are masters at it. They instinctively know other kids' vulnerabilities. There was this one boy . . . " Floyd stopped abruptly. He looked away from us and rubbed his chin.

"What is it, Floyd?" Lars asked.

Floyd hesitated before responding. "I guess it's okay," he said, speaking more to himself than us.

"Does this have something to do with the murder?" I asked.

"I don't know. I guess it does. The kid who just popped into my head, the one who was a master at setting up other kids. It was Kevin Landry."

No one spoke for a minute. I was the first to break the silence. "Was Kevin the kid being discussed at the clinical review?"

"No. Not that we hadn't discussed Kevin. Many hours have been spent trying to figure out an effective intervention for him. The boy we were reviewing that day was different in a couple of ways. Staff called Kevin the 'stealth provoker.' He would manage to get other kids to do things that would get them into trouble—pick a fight, violate a unit rule—without leaving a trace that he had been involved in any way. Most of the time the kid who had gotten into trouble didn't even realize Kevin had set him up. The other boy, I'll call him Jeff though that's not his real name, was just the opposite. He always got caught. Usually by the kids he was trying to set up, but also by the staff. Actually Jeff was much better off when the staff intervened; the kids usually pounded the hell out of him."

"Either he was not very competent or he wanted to be caught," Ollie observed.

"That's what Dr. Clover said at the review meeting," Floyd said. "She thought he had some kind of self-destructive urge. It made sense to me. Jeff didn't seem to get any satisfaction from setting up kids, even on the few occasions he was successful. He seemed genuinely sorry when staff pointed out to him what he had done. Kevin, on the other hand, got great pleasure from his accomplishments. He loved to see other kids pummel each other and he couldn't be happier when one of the boys was given a program restriction for an infraction Kevin had goaded him into."

"Not a very nice child," Lars said.

"Successful, though." Floyd realized at once what he had said. "At least he was until last week. He seemed to lead a charmed life. Usually a kid who causes a lot of trouble is given a few chances. If we can't modify his behavior after trying two or three interventions we usually find a way to discharge him."

"But I thought your program was designed for kids with behavior problems?" Ollie asked.

"It is. But we have our limits. When a kid disrupts our program too much we find a way to get rid of him. A kid can be real sick as long as his symptoms don't threaten staff or disrupt the unit program. Kids like Tommy are pretty sick but aren't a threat to the staff. On the other hand I've seen kids who caused a lot less damage than Kevin discharged abruptly. And they certainly hadn't achieved their treatment goals. For some reason the school tolerated Kevin's antics. Which is what made Jeff's clinical review so odd."

"How so?" I asked.

"After Jeff's therapist presented his case, Gloria Harrington gave a long speech about maintaining the integrity of the program and needing to set firm boundaries. She said that Possum Ridge was a treatment facility, but we couldn't help children who weren't motivated and we certainly couldn't tolerate a situation in which a child's safety was constantly being placed at risk."

"Meaning Jeff?" Ollie asked.

"I guess. She said we needed to seriously consider whether Jeff was appropriate for our program. She recommended that we notify his DSS worker and tell her to look for another placement for Jeff. Her comment struck me as odd for several reasons. First, the only person whose safety was at risk was Jeff. He certainly wasn't hurting other kids. I also was surprised that she was willing to give up his tuition payment, especially since Jeff didn't pose a real threat to the milieu. Our census has been shrinking during the past four years and it's no secret that Possum Ridge has big-time financial problems."

"How did the other staff respond to what Harrington said?" I asked, wondering what she hoped to gain by taking such a strong stand at a meeting which she usually didn't attend.

"Nobody said anything for a moment. I think they were too stunned. Then Dr. Clover responded. At first she was very polite and calm. She thanked Harrington for her report and told her that the safety of the milieu was certainly an important consideration in any clinical decision. Frankly, I think Doc was trying to blow her off. Harrington wouldn't give up though. She started getting personal. She questioned whether Jeff's therapist was on top of the situation and accused the staff of not intervening aggressively enough when there were early warning signs of potentially dangerous situations.

"Doc Clover is usually pretty cool. I've seen her diffuse some tough situations. But when Harrington said that Jeff was a troublemaker who should have been terminated from the program a long time ago, Doc lost her cool and laid into her.

"She said that Jeff's problem had very little to do with motivation, that he was a sick child who needed good psychiatric treatment, not moral persuasion. She told Harrington she wasn't qualified to make clinical judgments and ought to stick to pushing paper around her desk. Then she asked Harrington to leave so they could conduct their clinical review. Harrington looked like she was going to strangle Doc. She didn't do anything, though. Just gathered up her papers and left."

"So how come Dr. Clover is still at Possum Ridge?" I asked. "How come she didn't suffer the same fate as her husband?"

Floyd smiled. "You've seen Doc Clover?"

I nodded.

"Then you noticed a resemblance to another member of the Possum Ridge community."

"Prosic?"

"Yup. He's her brother."

We talked about the family connection and how Harrington must have sensed that even in his current condition Prosic wouldn't tolerate having his sister fired. Our server took our plates and asked if we were interested in having dessert. Lars ordered cannoli, Floyd had a huge slice of chocolate cake, and Ollie took our server's suggestion and got a rich-looking whipped cream and fruit concoction. I was so stuffed I could only manage a cup of coffee.

From the expression on their faces I surmised that the desserts were as delicious as the entrees. Ollie looked happy and I was glad for her. Looking at her still made my heart race but it was different now. I saw her beauty... and her intelligence and strength as well. But instead of my first thought being how Ollie would become part of my life, how we would be together for the rest of our lives, my reaction now was less intense, not quite as emotional. I still saw her as a special woman, someone I admired and wanted to know. Not as a lover though, but as... something else. What the something else was I didn't know, but it didn't seem quite as confusing as it had even a couple of days ago.

Our server brought the check and, true to form, handed it to Lars, gazing dreamily at him. He took the check without looking at her. I tried to pay for my dinner as well as Ollie's but he insisted on picking up the tab.

Floyd began to push back his chair but I wasn't finished with him yet.

"How about the other staff at Possum Ridge?" I asked. "Anyone unusual?"

"Nothing you wouldn't expect in that kind of setting." Floyd looked uncomfortable.

"How about the group we met in the parking lot? They struck me as pretty hostile."

"They're okay," Floyd said. "Grace is kind of insecure. Tries to prove she's one of the guys sometimes but she's kind of soft underneath. Does real well with the kids, especially the real sick ones."

That might be, I thought. But I had some doubt about how *real* Floyd was being at that moment. "How about Jack?" I asked. "Is he one of the better counselors?"

Floyd paused before responding. "No", he said softly. "Jack Liddy's not one of the better counselors."

"Anything I ought to know about Jack?" I asked, lowering my voice to match his.

"What do you mean?" he asked. From the worried tone of his voice I deduced that Floyd would not be a good poker player. I was fairly certain he knew what I meant. He glanced at his watch and turned to his uncle.

Before Floyd could speak, Lars shook his head and said, "This is not right, Floyd. If you know something that might help the young boy accused of killing that child, you need to tell Marty."

"Okay," Floyd said, exhaling sharply. "But I don't want anyone else to know I talked to you about this. You understand?"

I nodded. "I understand."

Floyd ran his hands through his hair and down his neck. "There've been rumors about Jack for a long time. At first I didn't pay any attention; Possum Ridge thrives on gossip. But one day I saw him with a short, heavyset man. It looked like they were involved in some kind of transaction."

"Drugs?" I said.

"That's what the rumors were. But I can't really say what was going on between Jack and the short, stocky guy. They were talking together in the parking lot, the one where the . . . uh . . . incident occurred this afternoon. They were standing about fifteen feet from my car. The short man had his back to me. I couldn't see what he was doing. As I approached my car I saw Jack hand something to the other man."

"What did it look like?" I asked. "Was it money? A package?"

Floyd shrugged. "I couldn't tell. It was small and it was hidden in his hand. When Jack saw me approaching he said something to the short man. He spoke softly so I couldn't hear him. Then he walked away."

"Doesn't sound unusual to me," Lars said. "The guy could've been scalping some UMass basketball tickets or something like that."

"That's what I thought at first," Floyd said. "Until I ran into Jack the next day in the cafeteria. He's not congenial, even at his best. But he was downright nasty to me that day. Told me to forget that I had seen him in the parking lot, that it was none of my business. He pointed his finger at me and said he didn't want it coming back to him that I'd been talking about him."

"So what did you do?" I asked.

"I told him not to point his finger at me."

"Why do you hang around with him?" Lars said. "He sounds like a real sleaze."

Floyd shrugged again. "We're not that close. Once a week a bunch of us go to lunch at the diner. My friend Eric works on the same unit as Jack. Sometimes he tags along. I never had any problems with Jack, at least until then. Since I told him to get his finger out of my face he's left me alone."

I still felt Floyd hadn't told us everything he knew about Jack. "What about the rumors? What were they about?"

"Nothing specific," Floyd said. "Just that Jack was involved with some of Northampton's less stellar citizens. If you wanted to score he could arrange it."

"Anyone else mentioned in those rumors?"

"No," Floyd said, shaking his head. "Not that I've heard."

"What about Dave?" I asked.

Floyd gave me a quizzical look. "Dave?"

"Yeah," I said. "Dave Porter. The guy who found Kevin's body."

"What makes you ask about him?" Floyd said nervously.

"I saw them together on my way to Dr. Clover's office. Jack was his usual charming self. Dave seemed nervous, kept looking at his watch. He couldn't wait to get away from me."

"I know that Dave and Jack work on the same unit. Once in awhile they hang out together. They're both pool freaks." Floyd looked at his watch, then smiled as he realized what he had done. "I'm not really trying to avoid your questions, he said. I'm supposed to meet my girl friend, Bonita. She doesn't appreciate it when I'm late."

Lars laughed. "He's right about that. Bonita has a clear sense of propriety. Punctuality is near the top of her list."

"You got that right, Uncle Lars," Floyd said, pushing back his chair. "When we were in college she would get up and leave class if the professor was more than five minutes late. She'd go straight to the Dean's office to complain. One time she demanded a partial tuition refund for our philosophy class because our teacher was chronically late."

"Didn't she ever hear of the fifteen-minute rule for full professors?" I joked.

"Not Bonita. She believes that etiquette does not recognize class boundaries. She would hold the Pope to the same standards she applies to a choir boy." Floyd stood. "I really have to go." It was more of a plea than a declaration. "You can call me if you have more questions."

Ollie had been quiet for awhile. Now she looked at Floyd and said, "Aren't you forgetting something?"

Floyd looked puzzled. "I don't know what you mean?"

"I think you do," Ollie said, turning her chair toward Floyd. "After Jack pointed his finger in your face, you didn't just let it go, did you? You were curious. You had to find out what he was into, what he didn't want you to know."

Floyd stood with his mouth open, staring at Ollie. "How . . . how did you know?"

"Just call it woman's intuition. So what did you find out about Jack?"

"Not that much. Just that he's partial to cocaine. Not heavy duty; more like a recreational user, mostly on weekends. Unfortunately he had a little problem with his cash flow. He got in a little too deep with his dealer, owed him more than two thousand dollars. The dealer gave him a choice: run a small franchise operation for him or let his associates use his knees for batting practice. Jack wasn't ready to give up deep knee bends."

"Who told you this?" I asked.

"My friend Eric."

"Was he with you this afternoon at the parking lot?" Ollie asked.

"Yeah, he was the other black guy."

"Did you find out anything else about Jack?" I asked.

"No, nothing," Floyd said, zipping up his windbreaker. "I've told you everything I know." He glanced at his watch. "I've really got to go. If I hear of anything, I'll let you know, Mr. Fenton. Just tell my uncle where I can reach you."

Floyd shook hands with everyone and thanked Lars for dinner. As he turned to leave, Ollie called to him. "Isn't there something else, Floyd?"

"What are you talking about?" Floyd said.

"Eric," Ollie said. "You haven't told us how he was involved with Jack."

Floyd stared at her again. This time he looked more puzzled than surprised. "What do you mean? Eric doesn't have anything to do with Jack. They work on the same unit, go to lunch together once in awhile. That's it, though. I don't know where you got that idea."

After Floyd left I frowned at Ollie. "You were guessing, weren't you?" I asked.

"What do you mean?" Ollie asked innocently.

"At first I was really impressed," I said. "When you pushed Floyd on what he did after Jack threatened him, I thought you were brilliant. Agatha Christie would have been proud of you."

Lars laughed. "Did you see Floyd's face when Ollie confronted him? His mouth was open so wide you could have dropped a whole salmon in it."

Ollie shrugged. "All part of an honest day's work."

"You should've quit while you were ahead." I reached over and poked Ollie lightly on her arm. Ollie looked down at where I had hit her, then looked up at me. I felt a twinge of anxiety in the pit of my stomach, but decided to stay on the offensive.

"Lars is right. You had Floyd in the palm of your hand. He probably thought you could read his mind. All you had to do was throw him a few open-ended questions and he would have opened his soul to you, told you everything he knew. You had the right idea when you asked if he had forgotten something. Then you went and spoiled it by getting specific. When you suggested Eric was involved with Jack, you not only shut Floyd down, you also lost your credibility with him."

Ollie stewed silently as I gloated. I knew I had been a bit harsh, but hadn't she asked for it? I didn't pass myself off as an art critic and certainly didn't pretend to be a bodybuilder. So why did Ollie think she could move into my territory? It wasn't right. I was pumping myself up pretty well and was about to continue my harangue when I noticed that Ollie was glaring at me. No sense pushing my luck. "At least you got some good information about snarling Jack."

Ollie smiled. "Even Miss Marple makes a mistake occasionally." She leaned across the table and punched me in the arm.

Her poke was not as gentle as mine.

I shook hands with Lars and thanked him for dinner. His grip was about as firm as it had been when we first met at Bart's. This time it didn't feel unfriendly. I turned to Ollie and put my hand on her shoulder. "I think we should talk."

She gave me a puzzled look then shrugged. "Okay. Let me say goodbye to Lars."

CHAPTER FIFTEEN

Sometimes I like school. It is mostly quiet and the teacher is nice to me. I don't like taking tests. They make me nervous. I like books. They smell good and the pictures are nice. I know how to read but I don't tell anybody.

The first thing Ollie noticed was the artwork. She complimented me on my choice of accommodations and suggested I consider applying for a part-time job at the Hotel and Convention Center if I needed extra money for my tuition payments.

Knowing that she was probably as uncomfortable as I was, I chose not to respond to her sarcastic comments. This took some self-restraint on my part, especially in light of my discovery and subsequent adjustment of the upside-down Picasso; but I didn't want to get into it with Ollie.

Not yet anyway.

"All kidding aside," I said, stuffing my dirty underwear into a plastic bag, "I was impressed by how you finessed Floyd into telling us about Jack's drug dealing."

Ollie looked at me quizzically, not certain whether I was being serious or just getting ready to challenge her investigative prowess again.

"I'm sorry I was so critical at the restaurant," I said. "To tell you the truth I was not only impressed but also a little envious of how you caught Floyd off guard."

Ollie shrugged and sat down in the upholstered chair. "Beginner's luck." I was about to disagree with her when she abruptly changed topics. "I know the last few days have been pretty tense between us, Marty. You haven't been too happy with the way I've acted and truthfully neither have I." Ollie looked down at her lap.

"I don't think you should . . . "

"Stop it!" she snapped. "You really piss me off when you do that. Can't you just let me say what I feel instead of making excuses for me or trying to chill me out? I don't need you to protect me, you know."

I certainly did know that. If I had any doubts, the incident at the school parking lot had erased them. "You're right about that. I do have trouble just listening to you, especially when you're talking about us. But that's not why I interrupted you this time."

Ollie folded her arms and gave me one of her 'this better be good' looks. "I'm all ears."

She wasn't making this easy for me.

"The truth is," I began, "You're not the only one having trouble with our relationship. For a long time I wanted to believe that your reluctance to commit to me was the only problem we had. Lately I've realized it's not that simple. I have my own doubts about whether we should be together."

Ollie unfolded her arms and sat on the edge of one of the beds. I walked over to the window. Looking out on the quiet parking lot I searched for inspiration but found none. I turned toward Ollie and took a deep breath. "I haven't been totally honest with you...or with myself. When I started graduate school I felt that I finally had some direction in my life, that I was entering the grownup world. Within the first couple of months I found myself thinking that it was time to settle down. If I could only find the right woman I would get married. Right after that I met you and immediately thought that you were the one."

"Swept you off your feet, didn't I?"

"Actually you did...in more ways than one."

"Let's not go there, Marty."

"Okay. At first I was really confused...and scared. All of my nice ideas about making a commitment, getting married and having a family were being put to a test, and I wasn't doing too well. But before long I began to calm down. I started to think of us as a couple and convinced myself that you were the woman I was supposed to marry. It all felt so perfect."

"We were a pretty good couple, for awhile."

"We were. I began making plans in my head. We would date for awhile then we might live together, but not for awhile. I didn't want to put too much pressure on our relationship. We would wait until I finished my thesis before getting engaged..."

"Sounds like you were doing some long-range planning."

"Yes, I was."

"Marty, that was a joke. Finishing your thesis, long-range planning."

"Oh. Yeah, I get it."

"I'm sorry. You were talking about getting engaged."

"About the time I began thinking it would be nice to have a summer wedding I realized that in spite of my grand plans for us, our relationship seemed to be getting worse rather than better. If I so much as mentioned that I was thinking about us beyond our next date you reacted as if I had dragged your family name through the mud and promised your first-born to the Colombian cartel."

"That's not fair, Marty."

"I know that now but I didn't then. As far as I was concerned I was Cupid and you were a curmudgeon. It wasn't until a couple of weeks ago I realized I was kidding myself." The shrill ring of the phone startled me. Who could be calling me at the motel? Gloria Harrington had called me earlier but there was no reason she would be calling again. I had given the answering service specific instructions not to give my mother this number. As I was reaching for the telephone it dawned on me that I had agreed to contact Faith Pasternak earlier that day. I must have sounded sheepish when I picked up the phone because Mrs. D asked if something was wrong because I didn't sound good. When I reassured her that everything was fine she broke into a hacking cough which went on for a full minute.

"Mr. Fenton," she gasped when her cough subsided, "your lawyer called."

"My lawyer? I don't have a lawyer."

I could hear her shuffling her message slips. "Let me see. Ah, here it is. The message reads 'Please tell Mr. Fenton that Faith Pasternak, the lawyer, called and ask him to return my call.' I guess I misquoted her."

I was beginning to rethink my position on cell phones.

I hung up the phone and returned my attention to Ollie. "Where was I?"

"You were kidding yourself."

"So I was. I was blaming you for not being accessible when actually I was the one who was questioning whether we were right for each other. More accurately, I began wondering whether I really wanted a long-term relationship with you. I realized that I had convinced myself that I was ready to make a commitment to you. Once I got to know you it was obvious that you are an intelligent, sensitive, attractive woman, highly desirable person, a perfect mate. As difficult as it was to accept, I finally came to terms with the painful truth. I was more in love with the idea of you than I was with you."

"How flattering. I've always wanted to be a lovable idea."

"I'm sorry, Ollie. I really am. I know it sounds awful and I'm a real asshole for deceiving both of us and even worse, trying to put the blame for our problems on you. The truth is I think you're a fantastic woman and wish I had the feelings I claimed I had for you..."

"Relax, Marty. As awful as your confession is, and I have to say it's one of the worst I've ever heard, I'm actually relieved. It makes it much easier to end our relationship, or should I say the illusion of our relationship. I don't have to feel guilty for breaking your heart and slowing down your quest for marital bliss."

"You're not mad at me?"

"More disappointed than mad. Though I resent the way you put all of this off on me. You acted like a real schmuck and I'm tempted to teach you a lesson." Ollie stood and took a step toward me.

"Hold on a second, "I said, raising my hands in front of my face and taking a step back.

Ollie lowered herself into a crouch and growled. Then she shook her head and began to laugh. "Not that kind of lesson, Marty. Some of us are not only more in touch with our feelings but have higher standards for how we treat people."

"Then what kind of lesson?" I still had my hands up.

Ollie looked at me with the crooked smile that told me she was enjoying my discomfort. "I haven't decided. I'll need to do some serious thinking to figure out a suitable response. The punishment should fit the crime. Isn't that what your law enforcement buddies say?" She turned, picked up her coat and headed toward the door.

"Wait a second. Shouldn't we talk about this more?"

"I think you've done plenty of talking for one night. I'm going to spend the night at Lars' place. He's got plenty of room. See you tomorrow, Marty"

It may have been my imagination but as she turned to walk out the door Ollie's smile seemed to grow into a full-fledged grin.

CHAPTER SIXTEEN

Everything should be in the right place. Socks and underpants in the top drawer. Shirts and sweaters in the second drawer. Pants in the bottom. Shoes go under my bed with my comic books.

A schmuck. I couldn't believe that Ollie had called me a schmuck. It was so unlike her. She rarely raised her voice and I had never heard her curse. She wasn't even Jewish. I wanted to convince her that she was wrong, to come up with a reasonable explanation for my behavior. But I couldn't.

I spent a half hour going over the reasons I had deceived Ollie and myself, and concluded that there weren't any good ones. The only consolation was that I had finally confronted the truth and confessed to Ollie. I should have felt better but I didn't. Even though I knew our relationship wasn't good for either of us it made me sad to think that I wouldn't be with Ollie anymore.

By that time it was too late to call Faith so I spent another few minutes feeling sorry for myself. Then I went to bed.

When I awoke the next morning, I was actually relieved that Ollie wasn't there. As difficult as it was to admit, I needed some space. At that moment it was easier to think about Tommy Hammond and the strange assortment of characters at Possum Ridge. I had neither the energy nor the will to wrestle with the thorny contours of our relationship.

After partaking of the motel's continental breakfast consisting of a weak cup of coffee and a stale Sara Lee Danish, I made a few telephone calls. I reached Larry Hammond at his office. He asked me how his son was and whether I had found anything that would clear Tommy. I filled him in on what I had been doing the past few days. I tried to strike a balance, giving him an honest account of what I had discovered without extinguishing the faint spark of hope that remained.

I was finding it difficult to produce enough promising information to kindle even a guardedly optimistic outlook.

Hammond thanked me for helping Tommy, which only made me feel more guilty. His voice was calm, as it always was, but there was something different about him. Several times he interrupted before I had finished. After I recounted Floyd's story about Jack's drug-dealing activities he apologetically asked me to repeat what I had said. He seemed distracted.

I asked if he and Mrs. Hammond were planning to come to western Massachusetts that day as they had initially told me. Hammond hesitated for a moment then said they had postponed their visit with Tommy until the weekend.

Reluctantly, I checked in with my answering service, which turned out to be a mistake on at least two counts. Mrs. D with her perennial cough and undying devotion to my mother was still on duty. I wondered if the woman ever slept and whether a few good nights of rest might rid her of that awful hacking. I listened to nearly two minutes of her cough-punctuated admonitions that I needed to give my mother more attention before I asked if I had any messages.

Which is when I received my second unwanted communication.

Professor Singleton had called to enquire about the status of my results chapter and to let me know he was looking forward to reading it over the weekend.

Fighting my urge to give up the telephone in favor of less painful modes of communication, I dialed Faith's office. My faith in Alexander Graham Bell's brain child was restored when Faith picked up on the second ring and told me she had visited Tommy again but he was no more responsive than he had been the first time. She said it must be awful to not be able to communicate with others. She said that people often told her they couldn't imagine how she coped with her handicap. Faith said that compared to Tommy her situation was a piece of cake. She also shared with me that she was petitioning the court to have Tommy moved to a forensic psychiatric program where he could receive appropriate care. Given the fact that Possum Ridge was the only treatment center in the area and it did not have a secure unit, she was not optimistic about the court granting her request. She said it made her feel better to be doing something even if it didn't produce any results. She told me her morning court appearance had been canceled and she would be happy to meet with me to review Tommy's case. If I left now I would have at least an hour to speak with Faith before my lunch meeting with Gloria Harrington.

On my way to Faith's office I made a mental list of possible suspects. My list included almost everyone I had met at Possum Ridge with the exception of Floyd and Bernard Washington. Even though Dr. Clover had told me Bernard was a former resident of Possum Ridge, I refused to believe someone who cared that much about kids could commit such a horrible crime.

It gave me a smidgen of satisfaction to narrow my list of suspects to seven, not counting the kids. On the other hand, my judgment has been known to be less than one hundred percent correct.

Faith was wearing a lavender silk blouse and a pale gray ankle-length skirt. They were good colors for her. She fixed me a cup of coffee, which was much better than the slop at the motel, and we settled in at her computer table.

"I put together a little chart," Faith said, booting up the computer. "Nothing fancy, just something to help us organize our thinking." She keyed in her password, clicked on a couple of icons, typed in a file name, and hit the *Enter* key. A grid appeared on screen. Along the vertical axis was a short list of names beginning with Tommy Hammond. At the top of the screen there was a series of row headings. At the left side of each column she had written a question: Relationship to Kevin? Reason to suspect? Possible motive? Access to Kevin? Alibi? Probability of being involved? Other questions that need to be answered? Sources of additional information? Most of the boxes contained one word responses such as yes, no or unsure. A few of the slots had more elaborate entries and some were blank.

"Pretty impressive," I said, scanning the grid.

Faith shrugged. "It's nothing, really. I'm a pretty compulsive person. Organizing things into an outline or table helps me to make sense of complex situations."

"Is that how you prepare a legal brief?"

Faith nodded. "Also how I plan my weekend chores."

"Maybe you can give me lessons. I haven't made it to the dry cleaners in six weeks." Finishing my thesis would have been a more relevant example, but I wasn't ready to reveal that vulnerability to Faith, at least not yet.

"As you can see I only have a few entries and even those aren't very complete. Can you add anything?"

We talked about the people on our list: Tommy, Dave Porter, the supervisor who found Kevin, Gloria Harrington, and Doctors Prosic and Clover. Other than Tommy, who had the misfortune to be sitting less than five feet away from Kevin's dead body holding a bloody knife in his hand, none of the other individuals on Faith's had any visible link to the crime.

I brought her up to date on my discussion with Floyd and added Jack and his cronies to the grid. "Not much of a list," I said. "Too many suspects, not enough evidence. Except against our client."

"I wouldn't want to be standing on the other side of the aisle trying to make a case against any of them. This would be a defense attorney's dream come true, if Tommy wasn't the client." Faith tapped several keys and the computer, sounding tired, whirred as it searched its memory. The computer wasn't the only one who was tired. The fruitless search for clues to clear Tommy and the tension with Ollie, not to mention the stress my unfinished thesis was causing, were taking their toll. I felt like I had just run a long-distance race on a hot summer day wearing a rubber raincoat.

Faith didn't look so great either.

Finally the whirring stopped and an unfamiliar document appeared on the monitor. "I have a few friends in the state A.G.'s office, Faith said. "Classmates from law school." She smiled briefly, then her face sagged. Good memories, painful memories. "Every once in awhile they'll help me out, especially if I sound pitiful, which isn't hard for me to do."

I wanted to say something, to tell her she shouldn't say things like that. To me she was far from pitiful. If anything, she was heroic.

But I couldn't find the right words.

"I was talking to one of my friends, an Assistant A.G. in the social services division. I told her I was involved in the Possum Ridge murder case. She asked me a few simple questions, then she fell silent. For a second I thought the line had gone dead. Then she told me it was odd that I was calling at that moment. I think she called it serendipitous. She said she had just received a report on another matter involving Possum Ridge. The report was confidential, but she trusted me and if I promised not to reveal the source she would send me a copy."

"Is that the document?" I said, pointing to the screen.

"Yes. I could tell she was pretty nervous about sending it to me when she said she would strap my skinny ass to my wheelchair and roll me over the edge of Mount Greylock if this ever came back on her."

The document on the screen was a memo from T. Flanagan, CPA, from the Office of the State Auditor to the Deputy Attorney General. The subject was an audit conducted in response to a concern raised by the state's residential child care licensing board.

"During an accreditation review site visit conducted last fall at Possum Ridge," Faith said, "the reviewer from the licensing board discovered a discrepancy between the number of children served by the school reported to the state in the year-end summary and the number listed in their student billing ledger at the facility. The reviewer stated that she probably wouldn't have thought much of it, but when she mentioned the discrepancy to the assistant director she became quite agitated and defensive. The accreditation reviewer decided this was outside of her bailiwick, so she told her supervisor, who reported it to the A.G.'s office. That's when Mr. Flanagan was brought in."

"And he paid a visit to Possum Ridge."

"That's right. Flanagan examined their student enrollment documents as well as their fiscal records and interviewed staff in both departments. He confirmed that there were discrepancies. Some children whose names appeared on the billing log were not on the enrollment list."

"Sounds fishy."

"That's what Mr. Flanagan thought." Faith pointed to the computer screen. "As you can see, he's got some hypotheses about the discrepancies, and his list doesn't include clerical oversight as a possible explanation."

The memo was thorough. It described in detail the auditing procedures he followed as well as his findings and preliminary conclusions. In the final paragraph he concluded there was sufficient evidence to warrant further action. He recommended that the state police be brought in to impound the school's records and conduct a formal investigation.

My brain processed this information and moved quickly to a new line of reasoning.

But Faith was already there. "What could Kevin Landry or Tommy Hammond possibly have to do with an enrollment scam?"

"Beats the heck out of me. But I'm certainly going to try to find out when I have lunch with Gloria Harrington." I glanced at my watch. "I better leave soon. I'm supposed to meet her in a half hour."

"Be careful, Marty. She may not be aware that the A.G.'s office is on to them. The last thing we need is to foul up their investigation. Obstruction of justice will be the least of our worries if my friend in the A.G.'s office finds out the confidential memo she shared with me was responsible for compromising their probe."

"Don't worry." I held up my hands. "Subtle is my middle name. By the way, when was that memo written?"

Faith scrolled up to the beginning of the memo. "Flanagan wrote the memo the day before yesterday."

"So it's possible the state police haven't begun their investigation yet."

"It's difficult to say. They can move pretty quickly, especially when there's a lot at stake. And I don't just mean money. The state agencies responsible for children's services have been hit pretty hard lately. There have been a rash of serious child-abuse incidents in foster homes that a lot of folks, including the media, attribute to bad judgment and insufficient monitoring by DSS personnel. And Medicaid has been under attack for the huge cost increase in kids' services this year."

"So what does that have to do with the state police?"

"A lot," Faith said as she deleted Flanagan's memo. "The governor is up for reelection. His opponent has been pounding on him pretty hard for his weak leadership. She accused the governor of being soft on crime and challenged him to refute the charge that he was letting state government 'go to hell in a hand basket.' If the governor is able to uncover and successfully prosecute fraud at Possum Ridge it will earn him more than a few votes from the citizens of the Commonwealth."

"Once again the demon politics raises its ugly head."

Something about my response seemed to catch Faith's attention. She looked at me for a moment, absentmindedly stroking her chin. Then she pivoted her chair and, muttering something that sounded like "son of a bitch," she reached for the telephone and punched in enough numbers to let me know she was making a long-distance call.

Not only was I at a disadvantage because I couldn't hear the person at the other end of the line, but the fact that Faith spoke in little more than a whisper made it difficult to know what the conversation was about. What I did know was that Faith was not inquiring about the health and well-being of the person to whom she was speaking.

"I must have been born yesterday," she said, slamming down the phone. "I really believed my so-called friend in the A.G.'s office was doing me a favor by sharing the Possum Ridge material with me."

"She wasn't?"

"Hell, no. She was using me. When I told her we were involved in the Landry murder, she saw a great opportunity to get us to do some of their basic investigative legwork without the state spending taxpayers' money—or more important, without them risking exposure."

"What do you mean?"

"Government agencies play by their own unique set of rules. In their game it's more important to avoid culpability than to achieve success. Making an error or even the appearance of doing something wrong will cost you a lot of points. Making a valiant effort but falling short of the mark puts nothing on your score card. You may even lose some points."

"So how do you win the game?"

"You don't. You just try to stay in it until you're sixty-five or the government has a fiscal crisis and offers an early retirement incentive to reduce their payroll. A few people, mostly high-level political appointees, think they can make a big score by overhauling an agency or promoting a major reform, but they usually underestimate the power of the system to maintain its status quo. The career bureaucrats know that if they're patient, the latest champion of the people will realize the system isn't going to change and will learn to play by the rules or take a high-paying job in the private sector."

"Not a big fan of government, are you?"

Faith chuckled. "Let's just say that I've spent a lot of time on the other side of the aisle representing people who've not been treated well by the Commonwealth or the feds. And I'm not talking about criminals. You better go. Don't want to be late for your lunch date with Ms. Harrington. Why don't we meet back here at four? I want to look at the medical examiner's report and speak to a few people I know who may have some insight into what's happening at Possum Ridge."

"Okay. We can certainly use some insight. But before I go you've got to tell me what the associate A.G. said when you called a moment ago."

Faith shook her head. "You really are a detective. Not happy unless you know every little detail."

"My friends in clinical psychology have another name for those symptoms: obsessive-compulsive disorder."

"I like detective better. More Hercule Poirot than Mike Hammer, but definitely the genuine article."

"Thank you." I felt flattered and embarrassed at once. The only person who compared me to other investigators was my lieutenant friend, Lou DeSantis, and his references were almost always tinged with a healthy dose of sarcasm. "As you were saying?"

"Alright. The witness will answer your question. My so-called friend, being the good bureaucrat that she is, told me she could neither affirm nor deny my allegation. Being the good lawyer and all around smart ass she is, she added that I couldn't prove it in a court of law."

"To which you replied?"

"I told her that if she ever tried to set me up again I would wheel my skinny ass down to her office and beat her ample ass to a pulp."

"What was her response?"

"She laughed so hard she nearly choked."

CHAPTER SEVENTEEN

Mommy and daddy haven't visited for a long time. Maybe they're mad at me. Mostly I'm good but sometimes I can't help it. Like when Kevin took my Game Boy and wouldn't give it back.

The drive to the diner was pleasant. The road climbed over a series of sloping hills, then crossed a stretch of well-tended farmland before ascending a steep incline that some easterners might have euphemistically called a small mountain. The trees were thick and the houses were sparse.

I wondered what it would be like to live in such a tranquil setting and I wondered how a place such as Possum Ridge, surrounded by such beauty, established for the purpose of helping those in need, could contain so much evil and corruption. The unholy trinity: drugs, death, and deceit. What could have happened to turn the place sour?

In spite of its rustic setting, the diner's parking lot was nearly full. Either a good sign or the only game in town.

I was greeted at the door by a gray-haired man with a thick Greek accent. I told him I was meeting Gloria Harrington. He said he knew Ms. Harrington well and she had not yet arrived. He showed me to the only empty booth in the restaurant, handed me a menu, and told me he would bring Ms. Harrington to my table as soon as she came in.

Looking around the diner, I was relieved that I did not recognize anyone from Possum Ridge. The last thing I needed was another confrontation with Jack and his gang, especially without Ollie's assistance.

Like all diner menus this one was huge. I tend to be health-conscious in my eating habits. When I go to a diner, however, I forget about fat and cholesterol and order grease and junk food. Sliced beef slathered with thick brown gravy accompanied by French fries and butter-drenched green beans are my favorites. I always save room for a thick slice of chocolate fudge cake and a scoop of vanilla ice cream, of course.

Growing up in New Jersey I had a large selection of diners to choose from. Some, like this one, were small and unpretentious. Others were enormous and gaudy, bearing faint resemblance to traditional diners. In a few towns, fierce competition had driven proprietors to build bigger and more elaborate structures, some of which resembled the Taj Mahal.

I consider myself somewhat of a connoisseur but I haven't discovered any relationship between the appearance of a diner and the quality of its cuisine. In fact, I had found that the only reliable indicator of whether the food is good is the taste and texture of the French fries. I look for thick slices of Long Island white potatoes cooked in extremely hot oil long enough to be crunchy, but not too dry. Undercooking is also a problem. Soggy spuds are a bad sign. My friends tell me if I want good French fries I should go to McDonalds. Most of them have grown up on fast food and don't appreciate the finer things in life.

Looking at the menu made me hungry but I decided it wouldn't be proper to order before Gloria Harrington arrived, even if she was late. When another fifteen minutes passed my restraint began to dissolve. Just as I was about to wave to the server, Gloria flew through the front door and scanned the dining room. She spotted me and hurried over to my booth. She was wearing a black blazer over a snug fitting, low scoop-neck red dress.

As she slid into the booth I got a whiff of a strong perfume that I hadn't noticed the last time we met. "I'm terribly sorry." She paused, trying to catch her breath. "We had an unexpected occurrence just before I was supposed to leave. Unfortunately it fell within my list of duties."

What sort of unexpected occurrence? I wondered. A drug deal gone bad? Another child murdered? A visit from the state police? Judging from the range of activities of Possum Ridge, her job description must have been very comprehensive. "I hope it wasn't anything serious."

"No, just a little misunderstanding about school policy. Staff are sometimes too creative in their interpretation of the rules."

Although I was curious to know whether selling drugs on campus fell into that category it was apparent that she wasn't interested in discussing the unexpected occurrence. "What's good here?"

"Almost everything. I'm partial to the souvlaki. The marinade is extraordinary."

I might have followed her suggestion but the ambiance of the diner had stimulated my appetite for cholesterol. "Bacon cheeseburger, fries, and a chocolate milkshake," I replied when the server requested my order.

We exchanged small talk for a few minutes before getting down to business. I learned that she had grown up in a small town east of Springfield. She had gone to U-Mass wanting to be a biochemist, but after two frustrating semesters gave up on that career aspiration and took a leave of absence from the university. She got a job as a receptionist at Possum Ridge and had been there ever since with the exception of a couple of educational leaves. To her credit she had earned a bachelor's and master's degree while virtually working full-time and had moved up more than a few notches on the administrative hierarchy in the process.

She seemed interested in my career. I wasn't proud enough of my vocational path to want to share it with her. Achieving the status of third-year graduate student in psychology at the age of thirty-eight with slightly more than three hundred dollars in my annuity account didn't exactly qualify me as a candidate for *People* magazine. Besides, I was growing impatient. What was so important that Gloria Harrington had to bring me to this out-of-the-way diner to tell me?

She must have sensed my impatience. Before I had a chance to redirect the conversation, she brought us back to the point of our meeting. "Mr. Fenton, it's obvious that you're a perceptive man." As she spoke she tugged at the strap of her dress, giving me a glimpse of her bra. The black lace of her undergarment created a nice contrast to her red dress. "I'm certain you couldn't help noticing that Dr. Prosic is . . . how can I put this . . . not functioning at an optimal level."

"Not to be disrespectful, but it might be more accurate to say that the good doctor was completely out of it. He looked like he was operating in a different time zone."

"I don't want to engage in a semantic debate with you, Mr. Fenton. The point is that Dr. Prosic's ability to direct our complex institution has diminished in the past couple of years, which is unfortunate for him and everyone at Possum Ridge. As much as we try to compensate for his lapses, there is no way our facility can maintain the level of excellence we have been accustomed to without the strong leadership of our director."

I didn't know where she was going with this monologue, but I was willing to indulge her, at least a little while. "Dr. Prosic wasn't always like this?"

"No. He's a brilliant man. When he took over the directorship, almost twenty years ago, the place was in a shambles. He developed Possum Ridge into the premier residential treatment facility for seriously troubled kids in New England. At one time we were getting referrals from the most prominent psychiatrists in Boston, Providence, and Hartford. Occasionally we even got kids from New York City.

"In addition to being an excellent administrator, he's also an extraordinary clinician. Even after he became director, Dr. Prosic worked with the most difficult-to-treat children. He has an uncanny ability to assess what's happening with a child. Not just make a diagnosis, but understand what causes a youngster to choose a particular coping style; the worries and fears that cause them to withdraw as well as the latent strengths they can draw on to confront their problems and help them return to the mainstream.

"As a therapist he was able to establish an instant and profound rapport. Kids trusted him. They sensed that he accepted them for what they were, that he wouldn't demand anything from them they weren't able or willing to produce. And they knew he would never betray or hurt them, which for many of our kids was a first."

Harrington paused for a moment as the waitress served our food. Her souvlaki smelled wonderful but I still wouldn't have traded it for my greasy bacon cheeseburger. I took a big bite and savored the perfect blend of taste and texture, knowing that the gauge on my cholesterol meter was rising rapidly.

Harrington took a few pieces of souvlaki, then resumed her account of the rise and fall of Dr. Harold Prosic. She described his efforts to build a therapeutic milieu in which even the smallest event or interaction was intended to advance the child's treatment program. She recounted his battles with the accrediting agency to convince them of the value of his innovative therapy. At risk of losing accreditation because of the uniqueness of his programs, Prosic persuaded the reviewer to grant the facility probationary status.

Three years later the program principles Prosic had been espousing were incorporated into the accrediting body's standards and continue to be an integral component of the review guidelines.

Before turning to Prosic's decline, Harrington reached into her purse and pulled out a tissue. She dabbed the corner of her eye, then blew her nose. She either had a genuine affection for the man or was an accomplished actor.

At the time I was not prepared to make a judgment.

"Dr. Prosic's deterioration was gradual rather than sudden. Over the course of a few years he slowly withdrew from his former position of active leadership. His attention span dwindled and even the slightest deviation from his regular routine threw him into a state of confusion. During the first year most staff didn't notice the change. Whether they were inattentive or we did a good job of covering up his disability was a matter of considerable debate among our small inner circle of executive personnel who knew that he was becoming dysfunctional.

"Once staff became aware of Dr. Prosic's condition they had a field day analyzing the cause of his deterioration. In fact, they spent more time discussing his diagnostic status than trying to figure out what to do about the void in leadership at Possum Ridge."

Though she didn't say so, it was apparent that Harrington had stepped in to deal with that problem, which probably saved Possum Ridge from total collapse. Most of the mid-level managers had been at the school for years. According to Harrington they were, for the most part, a reliable and competent group. By maintaining the same basic operating structure and confining Prosic's contact with staff to memos and other written communication, they were able to keep the facility running.

"Dealing with the board of directors was apparently more problematic. Faced with the growing constraints of managed care and the reluctance of state and local governments to send children to other jurisdictions, the board was justifiably concerned about the fiscal health of the institution. They wanted to know how Prosic planned to respond to these changes and they wanted assurance that the leadership of Possum Ridge was capable of maintaining its fiscal and programmatic viability. Keeping the board informed and sustaining their confidence in light of Dr. Prosic's declining capacity was no easy task."

Although Harrington's account of Dr. Prosic and the dilemma of Possum Ridge was interesting, my patience was wearing thin. Knowing that the facility faced serious charges of financial impropriety dampened my sympathy for their fiscal problems. More to the point, I needed to find out who killed Kevin Landry. The evidence against my client was compelling. I hadn't yet found a plausible alternative or even a tangible clue that might create reasonable doubt that Tommy had done it. And time was running out.

Why had Harrington asked me to have lunch with her? Did she really have something to tell me or was this just a ploy to distract me? If it was a ploy, what did she want to keep me away from? Kevin's killer? The drug traffic at Possum Ridge? The student billing fraud? Or were all of these events related in some way?

Once again Harrington seemed to read my thoughts. "I didn't mean to bore you with all of this local history. I just thought it would provide a context for what I'm about to tell you."

"Which is?"

"There is one problem that we haven't been able to deal with effectively in the current situation. It's a problem that may have contributed to Tommy Hammond's tragic plight and I thought you had a right to know about it. It's a problem that could have been prevented, but without Dr. Prosic's leadership and, in this instance, his cooperation, we were unable to intervene."

She now had my full attention. "And what might this problem be?"

"I believe you spoke to Dr. Clover yesterday."

I nodded.

"She's an insightful and dynamic person, as well as being a well-trained physician. She went to medical school and did her residency at Yale. She is also, as you may have discovered, Dr. Prosic's sister."

I nodded again.

"I was right. You are a good detective," she said with a smile that appeared to be genuine. I might have been wrong, though. Flattery tends to cloud my vision. "Unfortunately," Harrington continued, "Dr.

Clover has some unorthodox ideas about treating children with severe psychopathology. She believes they are so removed from a state of normalcy—emotionally, behaviorally, socially, and biochemically—that only a drastic realignment of their entire life will allow them to recover."

"Doesn't sound unreasonable to me. Didn't you say a few minutes ago that her brother also had unique ideas about treatment?"

"Yes, but there's no comparison. Dr. Prosic worked within an established theoretical framework and used acceptable therapeutic techniques. His contribution lay in the manner in which he combined these methods with elements of the child's everyday milieu. If a child had a phobic reaction to going to sleep Dr. Prosic would enlist the assistance of other children, particularly those who were socially withdrawn. He would ask these children to sit with the frightened child and offer assurance in ways that gave comfort to both the giver and the recipient. The child with the phobia became desensitized to the bedtime situation and the helper gained much needed self-confidence while picking up some social skills. Dr. Prosic was a genius at capitalizing on the human resources available to him in developing effective treatment plans."

I noted with sadness that she consistently referred to Prosic in the past tense. I also noticed that her eyes were red. She took a sip of water before continuing. "His sister, on the other hand, goes beyond acceptable practice standards, in both her use of psychotherapeutic technique and psychopharmacological agents."

"Drugs?"

"Medication would be the appropriate lay term. She often gives psychotropic medication to children with challenging problems even though there have not been clinical trials to establish the efficacy and safety of the medication for that clinical population."

"Is she able to help the children she treated?"

Harrington paused briefly before responding. "In a few instances children appeared to improve. There were also some disastrous results. One child who was diagnosed as having Asperger's disorder, a mild form of autism, withdrew into a catatonic state after being treated by Dr. Clover."

"Didn't anybody do something? Take disciplinary action, report her to the Board of Medicine?"

"That's the problem. Dr. Prosic wouldn't allow any action to be taken. They're not especially fond of each other, at least they don't appear to be. But he's quite protective of her. In his mind she's a brilliant psychiatrist. Only a few of us at the school are aware of her questionable practices and we've been unable to convince Dr. Prosic that his sister is a dangerous woman."

"Can't you go around him and report her to one of the regulatory agencies?"

The look Harrington gave me communicated her response more clearly than any words might. Whether her reluctance to act came from fear or respect was not apparent. I had difficulty imagining her being worried about her job. From what I had seen, her position in the organization seemed quite secure. "I've spent some sleepless nights second-guessing myself. Could I have made a more convincing presentation to Dr. Prosic? Was there anything we would have done to persuade Dr. Clover to stop these questionable treatments?"

Her consternation seemed sincere, but there was something about her story that troubled me. At the moment, though, I couldn't put my finger on what it was. "There must be a particular reason you're telling me this," I said, hoping her response might at least help me understand what I should be looking for.

"You know that Dr. Clover is Tommy's therapist."

"Yes."

"Well, Tommy is one of the children she was treating with one of her unorthodox prescriptions." She paused, waiting for me to make a connection. I wasn't about to say anything yet. I wanted to see where she was going. How would this knowledge help me to prove that Tommy did not kill Kevin? Even if I wanted to respond, what would I say? I didn't have any idea what it had to do with my investigation.

Harrington leaned forward, waiting for my response. When I didn't say anything, she sat back in her chair. Clasping her hands on the table, she took a deep breath, perhaps a sigh, before speaking. "We're pretty sure Kevin's parents will come after us. Failure to supervise, neglect of a minor in our care. Something along those lines. Because Kevin was in the custody of DSS for cause—his father abused him since he was a toddler and his mother's a heroin addict—we're not sure how the court will view their claim. Social Services isn't likely to take any action, though we'll probably not see a child from that jurisdiction for a long time."

I didn't know where she was going with this but I was content to let her continue.

"Tommy's family is a different story. Although DSS serves as his custodian, that's a formality, strictly for funding purposes; a cruel and arcane practice, I might add."

You don't seem to have a problem taking their money, I thought. Nor do you treat it as a formality, judging from the stonewall treatment the Hammonds received when they tried to find out what was happening after Kevin's death.

"Right now," Harrington continued, "the Hammonds are absorbed with Tommy and what's going to happen to him. After his case is adjudicated I'm certain their attention will turn to Possum Ridge and who allowed this to happen. We knew Tommy was disturbed. How could we permit such a volatile child to be alone with another student? And with a lethal weapon?"

I was beginning to understand what she was trying to tell me but I still wasn't sure why. "You're concerned that the Hammonds might sue you?"

"Naturally we've considered our potential liability."

"I'm sure your attorney has advised you about not speaking to anyone who might be a plaintiff in such an action without counsel present."

"Of course."

"And that includes their representatives, which means me."

She nodded.

"So why are you telling me about what you consider to be inappropriate treatment of Tommy by your own psychiatrist? Do you think the Hammonds might forego legal action against Possum Ridge in favor of a suit against Dr. Clover? I know shrinks are supposed to have deep pockets but I doubt that you pay Clover enough to qualify her for *Forbes*' list of wealthiest persons, even in western Massachusetts."

Red splotches suddenly appeared on her throat. "Mr. Fenton, in spite of any negative image you may have of residential treatment facilities or specifically Possum Ridge, we are not all money-grubbing, ass-covering leeches who prey on the vulnerabilities of troubled children and their families and laugh all the way to the bank."

Harrington's voice had risen as she delivered this impassioned defense of residential providers. Several other diners glanced our way but quickly returned to their meals and conversations. "I'm prepared to believe that," I said softly. "But you'll have to give me some help. You need to give me more information, be more specific. Why is it important for me to know about Dr. Clover?"

She glared at me briefly before responding. I guessed there wouldn't be any more strap tugging for my benefit. "Your clients are going to suffer a lot before this is through. With the recent changes in the Massachusetts statutes Tommy will probably be tried as an adult. If he's lucky they'll reduce the charge to second-degree murder. If he's really lucky the judge will consider his mental status when he issues a sentence. Whatever the outcome is, Tommy won't be coming home for a long time. It's hard to know precisely what Tommy is feeling but you can be damn sure his parents will be going through hell."

She took a sip of water but her eyes didn't leave my face. "Despite what you think of me," she said, returning her glass to the table, "I am concerned about Tommy and his parents. I also accept our culpability in this. Possum Ridge must bear some responsibility for this tragedy. When we accepted Tommy we knew he was prone to violent outbreaks. We should have provided closer supervision."

Her words sounded right but the delivery was a little too polished, as if it had been rehearsed.

"We're conducting our own investigation of why appropriate supervision didn't occur. And we will take strong disciplinary action when we find out who was at fault. We realize, however, that this won't help the Hammonds, so we're interested in exploring how we might provide more concrete assistance. To be precise, as you requested, I'm telling you about Dr. Clover's highly questionable treatment of Tommy because they have a right to know that their child's violent behavior may have been, in part, triggered by her misguided interventions and I want to demonstrate our willingness to reach out, to work with them. You might call it a token of good faith."

"You might call it that." My temples began to throb and I knew I was about to lose it. "I call it insensitive and inappropriate. No, I call it bullshit and I can't believe you brought me out here to tell me this."

"Naturally the actual settlement would be handled by the attorneys," she said, apparently unfazed by my brief outburst. "I've been authorized to share this information with you, to put our offer to negotiate on the table. Nothing more. If you or the Hammonds wish to discuss specific terms you'll have to work through our attorney."

She thinks I'm trying to up the ante, I thought. She must think everyone's mind works like hers. The throbbing was becoming worse. I took a deep breath and slowly let it out. I wracked my brain, looking for a pleasant image to distract me. When it came into focus I smiled. The sight of the state police carting off Possum Ridge's records made me smile. I began to relax.

"Perhaps I need to heed my own advice," I said. "I'll try to be more specific. My job is to get information on how Kevin Landry died. Until I find definitive evidence to the contrary I will continue to operate on the assumption that Tommy is innocent. My sole focus is on exonerating him. Anything that interferes with this focus, including bogus settlement offers, I consider to be irrelevant and possibly suspect. Your assumption that Tommy killed Kevin is a distraction, at best. If you want to be helpful you can tell me about some of the folks at Possum Ridge."

Harrington shook her head. "I should be insulted by your accusations, but I'm not. In fact I'm amused. You are a loyal and dedicated investigator, though a foolish one if you think you can refute the evidence against Tommy. Anyone in particular you want to discuss?"

I knew who I wanted to talk about but decided to float a trial balloon first. "What can you tell me about Bernie Washington?"

"As I told you yesterday, he's fantastic with the kids. He can walk into the middle of a gang war and have them standing in a circle singing Kum Ba Ya in less than three minutes. I don't know much about what the rest of his life is like, but at work he's great. I could run the school with half as many staff if they were all as good as Bernie."

"I understand he was a resident at Possum Ridge."

"That's right," she said without hesitation. "You've obviously been doing your homework. Ordinarily we don't hire former students. It can become complicated. But in Bernie's case we made an exception. And we've never had reason to regret it."

"The fact that he resented being forced to spend several years at a residential facility doesn't interfere with his judgment or his ability to support the program?"

"On the contrary. Bernie can relate to what these kids are feeling. He's able to help them understand why they are here and what they can do to get out and return home as soon as possible."

Time to move on. "How about Jack Liddy?"

I thought I detected a flicker of surprise in her eyes but I wasn't certain. I was looking for a reaction after all.

"Jack's okay, He's no Bernie Washington but there aren't many in his league. Jack is reliable and loyal. Some think he's a little rough on the kids. Personally I've never seen him act outside the boundaries of the program protocol."

"Meaning?"

"Meaning he applies the behavior management guidelines consistently. He seeks assistance from his supervisor when appropriate, and doesn't abuse the kids."

I decided to up the ante. "Rumor has it that Jack deals drugs."

"What!"

"Which part didn't you understand?"

"Jack selling drugs. That's absurd. Where did you get that from?" Her reaction seemed a bit overdone to me but I didn't get a chance to find out. A loud beeping sound startled me. Harrington reached into her purse and pulled out a small black pager. She pressed a button and looked at the small screen. "Excuse me," she said, sliding out of the booth. She took a cell phone from her purse and stepped outside. After a minute she returned to the booth.

"Unfortunately they need me back at the school. I can't say I've enjoyed our conversation but I don't think you have either."

I suppressed my urge to ask whether it was another minor occurrence that beckoned her back to Possum Ridge. I had a strong hunch about what had precipitated her office to call her.

I had a short debate with myself on whether I should order dessert. The bacon cheeseburger had been filling, but how often did I get to eat at a diner? In the end I settled on a compromise.

I ordered apple pie, without ice cream.

As I savored my dessert I thought about Gloria Harrington. A complex and puzzling woman. I couldn't say that I liked her and I definitely didn't trust her. Even now I was hard-pressed to know which part of her account, if any, was credible. To believe that her disclosure about Dr. Clover was intended to help the Hammonds and not malign the psychiatrist was a stretch, especially in light of her hostile confrontation with Clover and her dismissal of Clover's husband.

She was convincing, though. Part of me wanted to believe that her willingness to accept responsibility for the school's role in Kevin's death was genuine and not a ploy to keep me away from other lines of inquiry.

Then there was the little matter of the discrepancy between the student billing records and the school's report to the state. Not that I expected her to make a full confession to me. It did cast a wide shadow of doubt on everything she said, however.

Still, there was a lot about her that I admired. Running a complex facility like Possum Ridge was a tough job under the best circumstances. To keep the school functioning when the director could barely remember his name took a lot of skill—and cunning.

That was the thing that worried me the most.

I finished the pie and paid my bill. As diners go it was pretty good: a seven or eight on a scale of ten. In the parking lot I reviewed my options. It was a little past three. I could return a little early to Faith's office or if I were really conscientious I could begin to write up the results section of my thesis. Or I could satisfy my curiosity.

It was no contest.

I took a right turn at the parking lot exit and made the short trip to Possum Ridge in less than ten minutes. As I turned into the driveway leading to the administration wing, I fully expected to see a state police car parked in front of the building.

To my surprise there was none.

I was even more surprised when I saw Faith Pasternak's large silver van parked directly in front of the building.

CHAPTER EIGHTEEN

Who is that? Who is in my room? I don't like anyone in my room. It scares me. Stay away from me.

U nusual groups fascinate me. Nothing holds my attention as well as observing the dynamics of a group of people with different backgrounds and interests interacting in a meeting or social setting. In fact, my interest in what happens when an unlikely collection of people is thrown together is probably the major reason I chose to study social psychology.

The group assembled in Harold Prosic's office that afternoon was unusual, even by my standards. Dr. Prosic sat behind his desk trying hard to focus on what was happening in the room. For the most part he was succeeding, though occasionally his attention drifted to his favorite spot on the ceiling. Gloria Harrington stood next to Prosic's desk, arms folded across her chest. Her posture was a curious mix of defiance and self-protection. When I entered the room she gave me a look that made her glare at the diner seem friendly by comparison.

Seated at a small conference table opposite Prosic's desk were two middle-aged men wearing expensive gray suits. The taller man had a full head of silver hair that he probably paid someone a lot of money to style. He wore a burgundy tie that was a shade darker than the complexion of his face at that moment. The other man obviously had not contributed as generously to the financial health of the tonsorial profession. The only hair on his head was a narrow strip above the nape of his neck that looked like it could be easily maintained by an occasional swipe of an electric razor. The shorter man wore thick wireless glasses that did not relieve his need to squint constantly as he tried to follow the conversation. In his hands he held a handsome leather portfolio and an expensive ball point pen.

In the middle of this gathering sat Faith Pasternak, looking quite pleased with herself. She smiled at me as I entered the room, but before she could introduce me the man with the crimson face pointed a finger at Dr. Prosic and said, "What the hell's going on here, Harold? You can't keep me in the dark, dammit. I have a right to know."

"Of course you have a right to know," Prosic replied, shifting his gaze from the ceiling to the man with the crimson face. "But I don't have the foggiest idea what you want to know. I've kept you briefed on everything that's happened at Possum Ridge." Prosic glanced at Harrington, looking for confirmation. Unlike our last visit, she did not seem inclined to help him. Instead she continued to glare at me.

Taking advantage of the break in conversation Faith jumped in. "I was hoping you would make your way back here," she said to me. "Marty, this is Ted Millinger and Lasher Fiske. Ted is an old friend of mine. He helped me get set up in my office after . . . the accident. He's also the chairman of the Possum Ridge Board of Directors. Lash is an esteemed colleague who represents the school in matters of the law." I waved awkwardly. They did not return my greeting, but Faith was not deterred. "Marty represents Tommy Hammond. He's a private investigator from Syracuse. He and I—mostly he—have been trying to find out what happened to Kevin Landry. Which is what brings us here."

"Hold on, Faith," the taller man said, raising his hand. "I need some answers, Harold. Faith tells me there's something fishy going on here. She's always been a straight shooter so I have no reason to doubt her. I need to know what's going on and why you haven't kept me informed. And your answers better be good or you're in deep trouble."

Prosic looked at Millinger like he was speaking a foreign language. "I wish I could help you, Ted, but I'm afraid I can't."

Millinger threw up his hands in frustration. Fiske jotted some notes in his portfolio. Prosic looked to Gloria Harrington for assistance but she didn't seem to notice. She was too busy shooting mental darts at me.

Faith continued to smile.

"Okay," Millinger said. "It looks like we're going to have to go into executive session." Turning to Faith he said, "You and Fenton will have to excuse us. Don't worry. I'll keep my end of the deal. I'll call you later."

"You'd better," Faith said. "I know where to find you." Blowing a kiss to Millinger, she turned her chair and rolled toward the door. I followed obediently.

I waited until we were outside. "Do you mind explaining that to me?"

"It's simple," Faith said, still smiling. "Ted and I negotiated a little agreement. I told him I knew something he couldn't afford not to know. Then I persuaded him to make some inquiries on our behalf in return for me telling him what he needed to know."

"What about your buddy in the A.G.'s office? Didn't she threaten you with bodily harm if you told anyone about the Possum Ridge investigation?"

"She did and I didn't."

"Huh?"

"I didn't tell Millinger about the auditors' findings or the state police investigation. I simply told him there was something rotten in Denmark and he would be well advised to consult with King Prosic."

"Literary references aside, aren't you worried about compromising their investigation?"

"I'm afraid it's too late for that."

"How do you know?"

"We lawyers aren't as unprincipled as you think. I called my friend in Boston to let her know what I had done. She told me the state police were given the green light this morning. They should be here any moment."

"You're living dangerously, counselor. Even if you didn't technically violate your oath of silence I can't imagine that your friend in the A.G.'s office is happy with you. I bet she could make things unpleasant for you."

"That thought crossed my mind," Faith said solemnly. Then she smiled. "Fortunately for me Audrey, my friend at the A.G.'s, is still capable of experiencing guilt. She felt so bad about tricking me into doing her legwork that she decided to overlook my indiscretion. She told me I was off the hook. I had no need to fear payback . . . this time."

"How about that. A lawyer with a conscience."

"Careful, Fenton," Faith said, pointing at me. She opened her briefcase and pulled out a thin manila folder. "My badgering finally paid off. The judge ordered a psychiatric exam for Tommy, at the county's expense. Darrow's really pissed. They brought in a prominent child psychiatrist from the medical school in Worcester. I've heard he charges three fifty an hour, including travel time."

"Isn't that what you charge?'

Faith gave me a nasty look. "The good news is he confirmed that Tommy has some heavy-duty psychiatric problems."

"That's the good news?"

"Yes. It gives us a strong basis for arguing that Tommy isn't responsible for his actions."

"And what's the bad news?"

"First, the psychiatrist concluded that Tommy is quite capable of committing a violent act. His disorder is characterized by an inability to control impulses and his case history is filled with examples of aggressive behavior. Second, Darrow is going to move to try Tommy as an adult."

"But he's only fourteen."

"Unfortunately the Commonwealth no longer acknowledges that chronological distinction. A few years ago Massachusetts tightened up the statutes on juvenile offenders. Under the new laws, persons between the ages of fourteen and seventeen charged with murder go directly to district court and are tried in accordance with usual criminal proceedings. The fact that Tommy allegedly killed Kevin while he was in a treatment facility won't help when the court considers whether he's amenable to rehabilitation."

"So, what can we do?"

Faith shrugged. "Our best bet is to prove that Tommy didn't kill Kevin. If we can't do that . . . I'm not sure. None of our options are very good."

Once again she looked small and frail, so unlike the dynamic woman-in-charge she appeared to be a few minutes ago in Prosic's office. Had she actually changed or was I projecting my own feelings of the moment onto her? "Well, we won't have to worry about our options." I was trying to convince myself as much as Faith. "I'm going to find out who killed Kevin. And when I do Tommy will be cleared."

Faith reached for my hand. "You're a good man, Marty Fenton.

If I were ten years younger, I might give your girlfriend a run for her money."

I blushed. Not just because of what she had said, but because I had entertained a similar fantasy. Except in my version her additional ten years weren't a factor.

Sensing my discomfort, Faith suggested we split up and pursue our separate lines of inquiry. She intended to consult with a colleague who was an expert on juvenile forensic law. She would call me when she heard from Millinger. My assignment, she said with a small grin, was to find Kevin's killer.

I told her that Tommy's parents were coming the next day. We agreed to meet with them in her office at noon. I walked with Faith to her van and watched her open the side door and lower the hydraulic lift. She held out her hand and I took it. To my surprise, she pulled me toward her and reached up to hug me. She had more strength than I expected and I lost my balance. Fortunately I was able to grab the arm rest on her chair before falling into her lap. She laughed heartily and squeezed me. I leaned over awkwardly and put my arms around her. Hugging Faith was certainly different from embracing Ollie. In spite of my tenuous position I relaxed and rested my head on her shoulder. I hadn't noticed before that Faith wore perfume, but now, with my nose buried in her neck, I noticed an alluring floral scent.

After a few seconds she released me and I pushed myself to an upright position. Neither of us spoke as she navigated her chair onto the lift and into the van. When she was settled behind the steering wheel she gave me a small wave and backed out of the parking space.

I watched her pull away from the administration building then walked to my car. As I turned onto the main road, I passed two large blue and gray sedans. Glancing in my rearview mirror I saw the state police cruisers turn into the driveway leading to Possum Ridge School.

CHAPTER NINETEEN

He's too close. I don't like the way he smells. Take a big breath.
Count to ten. Walk away. That's what Bernard tells me.

O n the drive back to Northampton I thought about my reaction to
Faith. I had no doubt that my affection for her was genuine. But
where had it come from? Her remark about giving Ollie a run for
her money had certainly struck a responsive chord. Though in all honesty,
I was attracted to Faith before she revealed her feelings. Was it some kind
of male guardian thing? Did her disability bring out a protective instinct
in me?

It was not the first time I had been attracted to a vulnerable woman.
Last year, when I was looking for Fred Majorski, a missing railroad
engineer, I found myself drawn to his frightened green-eyed daughter,
Janet. In many ways, that situation was more clear cut. Janet really was
dependent on me to find her father. Watching Faith handle the security
guard at the detention center and seeing her orchestrate the gathering at
Dr. Prosic's office would give pause to anyone inclined to characterize her
as vulnerable.

And what about Ollie? How would this theory of dependency apply
to her? I couldn't think of any woman who needed me to protect her less
than Ollie. Not just physically, either. I was the one constantly pressing
her for some kind of commitment. She seemed content with enjoying my
company with no need of assurance that our relationship would lead to
something permanent.

Come to think of it, Ollie and Faith were similar in many ways. Not
physically, of course, but in other respects. Both were women of strong
convictions, with a clear sense of right and wrong. While their styles were

different, both were assertive to the point of fearlessness. Ollie almost always got what she wanted, and from what I had seen, Faith seemed to be at least as successful.

So how did Janet Pafko fit into this dynamic?

Perhaps my graduate student friends in clinical psychology weren't so far off target when they told me I had about as much insight into my own behavior as a headless chicken.

Feeling resigned to the fact that I wasn't going to make sense of my preferences for women at that moment, I switched on the radio. Stephen Stills was belting out the lyrics to one of his classic hits from the seventies, the one whose chorus begins, "If you can't be with the one you love, love the one you're with."

Which didn't do anything for my current state of confusion.

I decided to stop by the college before returning to the motel. After hearing Ollie extol the virtues of her alma mater I was curious to see Smith College. At this rate it didn't seem likely she would be showing me the campus. So I decided to take my own self-guided tour. Taking a walk might be good for my head.

Finding a parking space was tough, but the rest of my tour was pleasant. Ollie was right about the campus. With its old stone and brick buildings scattered throughout the park-like setting designed by Frederick Olmsted, best known as the architect of New York's Central Park, it was an ideal setting for contemplating the wonders of nature, reading poetry, or throwing a Frisbee. I especially liked the Japanese garden and the path along the narrow river that seemed to go on forever.

I had hoped to sort out my confused feelings about Ollie and Faith in this pastoral setting. Unfortunately my stroll through the beautiful campus did little to clear my mind. After thirty minutes I gave up and decided to return to the aesthetically inferior surroundings of my motel.

The desk clerk greeted me with a smile and a small stack of messages. Consistent with its uncluttered decor and rustic ambiance, the motel had neither voice mail nor message lights on the room phones. Guests wishing to know whether anyone was interested in communicating with them had to either call or stop by the front desk. Unless, of course, one happened to carry a pager, cell phone, lap top computer, or some other electronic device designed to keep you from paying attention to your immediate environment.

Most people would consider the primitive communication arrangements of the motel to be inconvenient at best. With my aversion to answering machines and other forms of impersonal communication, I found the old-fashioned message system refreshing.

I sorted through the scraps of paper, discarding those that simply conveyed information. Ollie was going to sit in on one of Lars' evening studio classes. She would call later. Larry Hammond had called to confirm they would be arriving in Northampton later that night. He left the telephone number of their motel and asked me to call him in the morning.

The other messages requested a response. My answering service let me know that my mother had asked them to contact me. It wasn't exactly an emergency, but if I really loved her, I would call right away or even sooner. Lou DeSantis asked me to call him when I had a moment. He had some interesting information for me. The last message was unexpected and even more compelling than Lou's cryptic teaser.

I thanked the clerk for the messages and walked quickly to my room, anxious to satisfy my curiosity.

She picked up the phone after the first ring. "I'm sorry to be late in the getting back to you," I said.

"Would it be possible for you to meet with me within the next half hour?"

"Sure. Where do you want to meet?"

"How about my office?"

"That would be fine. I can be there in twenty minutes."

"Good. I'll be waiting for you."

I hung up and started to leave, but before I got to the door the phone rang. It was the desk clerk, who cheerfully informed me that while I was on the line I had received another call. The caller hadn't left her name but said she would try again in a few minutes.

I guess I'm kind of old-fashioned in some ways. When someone says they are going to call at a specified time, I feel it's important to be available to receive that call. Having been burned by telephone solicitors whose message promised me their next call would bring me substantial benefits, I had become more wary. Still, in most instances I succumbed to my sense of proper telephone etiquette.

This time the decision to wait was even more complicated. I had another commitment, one I had personally made. Waiting for this unidentified caller would likely interfere with my ability to meet this obligation.

I struggled briefly with my dilemma and reached a compromise that allowed me to reconcile my ambivalence, at least for the moment. I would wait five minutes. If the call hadn't come by then I would ask the desk clerk to get the caller's name and number. If I drove above the speed limit I could still be on time for my meeting.

Four minutes later the phone rang. Faith apologized for not leaving more information. She had to make an important call to a client and didn't want me to be frustrated by reaching a busy signal. My pleasure in finding another person who didn't subscribe to call waiting outweighed the anxiety her anonymous message had caused. I forgave her.

It was odd speaking to Faith on the phone after our intimate encounter in the school parking lot. I wanted to say something to her but was having trouble finding words. I wasn't clear enough in my own mind. I was also afraid she might take it the wrong way, that it might interfere with our ability to work together on Tommy's behalf, which had to be our first priority now.

For whatever reason, Faith also chose not to discuss our sudden display of affection. Perhaps there would be a better time. Perhaps.

She reported that Ted Millinger had called to brief her on his discussion with Prosic and Harrington. He hadn't learned much, their conversation having been interrupted by the arrival of the state police, but there were a few things he was able to tell her. First, it was obvious that the school's financial situation was a disaster. Dr. Prosic didn't seem to have any real awareness of what was happening beyond knowing that enrollment was down and they probably wouldn't meet their revenue projections. Harrington had been predictably vague, but when pressed, had acknowledged there had been some mismanagement of funds. She did not provide any details. Whether she was unwilling or unable to elaborate was not clear, though Millinger was inclined to believe she damn well knew what was going on and had probably played a key role in any improprieties that may have occurred. As for Prosic, it was Millinger's best guess that he didn't have a clue about what was going on around him.

The only thing that was clear, according to Millinger, was Possum Ridge would be embroiled in a long series of investigations and judicial processes that would significantly alter and might possibly destroy the institution.

When Faith had finished recounting Millinger's description of the school's legal woes I asked, "What about Tommy? Did he learn anything about Kevin's murder?"

"He asked Prosic and Harrington about it. Prosic barely remembered the incident. At first Harrington was evasive but eventually told him she wondered whether Dr. Clover's unorthodox medical management of Tommy might have been a contributing factor. According to Ted, she was reluctant to say much about it."

"Maybe because Clover is Prosic's sister."

"Could be. Whatever the reason, she didn't elaborate."

I was disappointed in her report. "Seems like we got the short end of the deal. Millinger got some advance warning of the state police raid and we didn't learn anything new."

"It looks that way, but there was no way of knowing beforehand. Besides, Ted is a good friend. I felt I owed it to him. I'm sorry."

"Hey, I wasn't blaming you." I was suddenly aware that her reaction to my disappointed tone might have been triggered by factors beyond our professional relationship. "Speaking to Millinger was a good idea, an excellent idea. He might have been able to squeeze something out of them that we couldn't have gotten. It's not your fault that it didn't work. You did what you could."

There was a brief pause on the other end of the line. "I said I was sorry, Marty, not devastated." She spoke without inflection so I couldn't tell if she was irritated or amused. I thought it best not to ask.

"What happens now?" I asked. "With the state police, I mean."

"They'll impound all of the administrative records: billing information, revenue receipts, enrollment data. Probably haul it to the regional headquarters for safekeeping. First thing next week the team from the A.G.'s office will pore over the documents. If they think there's sufficient evidence of a violation, they'll move for an indictment."

"How long will it take?"

"The initial phase will move pretty quickly, probably no more than a few weeks. Once it's established that this is an indictable offense and specific individuals are charged it may take as much as a year before they go to trial. The wheels of justice don't move as swiftly as advertised."

"And if they don't find sufficient evidence?"

"From what I've gleaned Possum Ridge is emitting a pretty foul odor. The state's not likely to walk away from this, even if they don't find a smoking gun. They'll be all over the school like nerds on the internet."

"Haven't heard that one before."

"It's not original. My nephew told me. He has a computer mouse grafted to his palm."

"How will they be 'all over' Possum Ridge?"

"The state has many ways to make an organization's life miserable: auditors, licensing agencies, consumer protection boards, not to mention the tax department and the many branches of the attorney general's office responsible for assuring compliance with numerous sections of the code of the Commonwealth of Massachusetts. And if that's not enough, you can bet that the Justice Department agencies will quickly develop a keen interest in the Possum Ridge School. Which reminds me, Ted told me Harrington did pass on one choice piece of information to him."

"Anything to do with Tommy?"

"Hard to tell. It doesn't appear to be relevant, but we shouldn't rule it out. Harrington mentioned that she recently had a visit from a couple of members of DEA, the federal Drug Enforcement Agency. They asked some questions about a few staff members, but didn't tell her why they were asking."

"Did she tell Millinger the names of the staff?"

"Not at first. But Ted coaxed it out of her. I told you, he's a good friend."

"And?"

"And he gave me two names. The first won't surprise you: Jack Liddy. The second name was one I wouldn't have guessed."

"Do you enjoy stringing me along?"

"You're a detective. You're supposed to like mystery and suspense."

"Only in moderation. Right now I've got more than my fair share of unanswered questions."

"Okay. The DEA is interested in none other than the good Doctor Clover."

Too many unanswered questions. An understatement if I ever uttered one. As I drove to my appointment, for which I would definitely be late, I wrestled with one of those unanswered questions, the most recent one to plague my brain: Was the DEA really interested in Dr. Clover, or had Gloria Harrington fabricated this story to get back at her archenemy? Or even worse, had she actually met with the DEA and offered Clover to them as someone they should suspect?

The fact that she mentioned Jack did not make it easier to answer this question. Given Floyd's account of Jack's involvement with drugs, it was possible that the DEA would have knowledge of his illicit activity. Though why they would be interested in such a small-time player was another question I couldn't answer. Unless they wanted to use him to get to a heavier hitter.

On the other hand, Jack's high-profile dope activity could just as easily be used to support the argument that Harrington had made up the whole story about the DEA. If Floyd knew about Jack's drug dealing, it was likely that Harrington would also have this knowledge.

The question of whether Dr. Clover was on the DEA's list of prime suspects was beginning to give me a headache. My only consolation was that in a few minutes I would have an opportunity to address that question directly.

The campus looked good in the light of the full moon. The rustic cedar-sided buildings, bordered on the back by sprawling lawns and surrounded by a thick forest of hardwoods and evergreens, exuded tranquility. It was hard to believe so much distress and ill will resided on these premises. Both within the children and in the institution itself.

A pale light illuminated the window of Dr. Clover's office. I climbed the stairs and knocked on her door. I heard a scraping sound, a chair being moved, followed by heavy footsteps. The door was pulled open and Dr. Clover stepped forward. She was dressed as she had been when we met the day before: dark tailored suit, white shirt, vest, and tie. She extended her hand and shook mine firmly, but offered no other greeting. I followed her into her office where she sat behind her desk and motioned for me to sit in one of the two chairs facing her desk.

It wasn't until she pointed to the chair that I noticed the other chair was occupied. Looking up at me was the snarly face of Jack Liddy.

Only this time he looked more frightened than mean.

"Don't worry, Mr. Fenton," Dr. Clover said. "I asked Jack to join us. He needs your help, as do I."

I looked over at Jack. He seemed smaller than I remembered, and less menacing. Studying his face, I wondered if the fear had been there all along. Had my own feeling of intimidation prevented me from seeing it?

"What about it, Jack?" I asked. "You want my help?"

Jack winced. I pride myself on asking probing questions, but didn't consider this one to be in the intensely painful range. Jack glanced at Dr. Clover. She raised her eyebrows and gave him a slight nod.

"Yeah," he said softly, "I guess so." I was not at risk of being bowled over by his enthusiasm.

"So, how can I help you?"

Dr. Clover tapped her fingers on the desk. "I know you haven't been getting much cooperation from Possum Ridge staff. It must be frustrating." I was immediately suspicious. This was not the same hard-nosed, stick-to-the-facts scientist I had previously encountered. Either she was softening me up for a big favor or . . . I couldn't think of another reason for her empathic approach. "Institutions like Possum Ridge tend to close ranks during a crisis," she continued. "Everyone comes together to fend off the outsiders. It's a strange phenomenon. Even staff who can't stand each other, who would just as soon tear each other's eyes out as offer a civil greeting, band together to protect the institution."

"Sounds like a territorial instinct," I said. I was tempted to challenge her institutional bonding theory, based on Gloria Harrington's eagerness to implicate her in every bad deed that occurred at the school, but decided to put off that discussion until later.

"You might call it that. I couldn't say for sure. I'm a psychiatrist, not an anthropologist, as you know." Dr. Clover, the empiricist, had returned. "I apologize for the stonewalling you've received," she continued, "Though to be fair, most of us, including me, didn't know anything about Kevin's murder or Tommy's possible involvement. At least not until today."

"And what happened today?" I said impatiently.

"A couple of hours ago, Jack came to my office and told me some disturbing things about Kevin's death." She shifted her attention to Jack, who looked as if he wanted to slide under the desk. "I think it would be better if you told Mr. Fenton what you know."

Jack winced again. He clearly had a low threshold for pain. "I didn't have anything to do with killing Kevin," he blurted out. I waited for him to elaborate but he said nothing.

"Let me give you some background," Clover said after a moment. "Would that be all right, Jack?"

I didn't have to look over to know which way his head was moving.

Dr. Clover shifted in her chair before speaking. "Earlier this afternoon Jack came to my office. He was rather agitated. He told me he had just seen two state police cars and was afraid they might be coming for him. He didn't know what to do and wanted my advice. I asked him why he thought the police might be coming for him and he told me he was involved with some people who had something to do with Kevin's death."

"Involved?" I asked.

Dr. Clover and Jack exchanged glances before she responded. "I realize there is no provision for confidentiality in this conversation since neither of us is your client. I would be appreciative if you would treat what we're about to tell you with discretion."

"I can't promise you anything. If I hear something that will help my client I'll use it. Tommy's well-being is my first responsibility."

"As it is mine," Clover said.

"Short of anything that has direct bearing on Tommy, I'll take your request for discretion into account."

"Fair enough," she said, not even bothering to confer with Jack. "Jack has been foolish enough to become involved in the sale of illicit drugs. Mostly small transactions involving marijuana and cocaine. He sells to people in neighboring towns and, I'm sorry to say, occasionally to staff at Possum Ridge."

"How about the kids at the school?"

Jack shook his head vigorously.

"According to Jack," Clover continued, "until recently, he worked for some people from Springfield. A couple of months ago, a more powerful group moved into this area. There were some messy negotiations resulting in a few dead people and eventually the new group displaced the old one. Because they didn't have any contacts in this part of the Pioneer Valley, they approached Jack. He says he didn't have much choice, though I'm not sure I agree."

"Where is the new group based?" I asked.

Dr. Clover gestured to Jack, who said, "New York."

"Where in New York?"

"Upstate. Utica and Syracuse."

Wheels began to turn rapidly in my head.

CHAPTER TWENTY

Why do they keep asking me what happened to Kevin?

For the next fifteen minutes Jack talked about the drug dealers from central New York, how they infiltrated the Pioneer Valley and the damage they had done since moving into the area. As a storyteller Jack would never be mistaken for John Grisham, but he provided a clear picture of what had occurred. What he lacked in eloquence, he made up for with his vivid description of the drug dealers' ruthless treatment of those who attempted to interfere with their entrepreneurial endeavors.

By the time Jack had completed his account I had a pretty good sense of what had happened to Kevin.

I knew why he had been murdered and how his life had been taken. Most important, I knew that Tommy had not stabbed Kevin. His murder had been premeditated and was accomplished with cold-blooded efficiency by a member of the drug gang. Jack said he didn't know who had actually stabbed Kevin, but he heard from one of the dealers that it had been someone fairly high in the organization's hierarchy. He also was told his own life would be in jeopardy if he shared this information with anyone.

In addition to not knowing who had actually killed Kevin, I was not clear how Tommy had been set up and I still didn't understand what role, if any, Dr. Clover had in this mess.

"Why did Jack come to you?" I asked.

Clover looked at Jack. "You can tell him," he said.

"I've known Jack for a long time. He trusts me . . . as much as Jack can trust anyone. When things bother him, he sometimes comes to see me."

"Jesus, Doc," Jack said impatiently. "Stop beating around the bush. I don't care if he knows you were my therapist."

It took a moment for me to process this information. Jack didn't strike me as a self-discloser. It was hard to imagine him sharing intimate secrets or expressing deep-seated fears to a psychiatrist. Still, I wouldn't want to underestimate Dr. Clover's therapeutic skills. I recalled my first meeting with her. Sitting in her office, I had felt her eyes boring into me, like a powerful magnet drawing from me feelings buried in the deep recesses of my mind.

"Were you a student here?" I asked Jack.

"No. I lived in town. I came to her office a couple of times a week for about a year."

I wanted to ask him what brought him into therapy, but I checked myself. Jack's treatment wasn't relevant to Tommy's current situation. Besides, if I was going to probe into Jack's therapy, I would rather know about the outcome. Judging from his current level of surliness, it was hard to imagine that he had benefited from treatment. If he had made progress, he must have been a real bear before he began therapy.

I turned my attention to Dr. Clover. "So Jack came to you because he was afraid he was going to be arrested?" She nodded, "And you advised him to tell me what happened." She nodded again. I looked at Jack. His lips were pressed, his brow furrowed. He was either concentrating intently on our conversation or experiencing severe intestinal distress.

"And what did you expect me to do?" I asked both of them.

They exchanged glances before Clover replied. "We thought you might use this information to help Tommy, to convince the authorities that he didn't kill Kevin."

"That's why you asked me to come tonight. For Tommy's benefit?"

"Yeah," Jack said. "To help the kid."

"Any other reason?" I asked.

Jack shrugged. "I figured the cops might go easy on me if I told someone what happened before I was collared. That way it wouldn't look like I was telling them all this just to save my ass."

"Very clever," I said. "But I'm not convinced."

Jack jumped up. "You don't believe me," he shouted.

I considered whether he might come after me. If circumstances were different, he probably would have thrown a few punches in my direction. But with Dr. Clover sitting behind her desk I guessed I was safe.

"Why don't you sit down?" I said softly. "It's not that I don't believe what you've told me. It's just that I don't think you're telling me everything."

Jack sat. "Okay. There is something else. These people I've told you about, they're brutal. If they even suspect that I've ratted them out they'll kill me. I wouldn't be any safer in prison than out here. They're very powerful and they don't let anything or anyone stand in their way. I figured if you told the cops what happened to Kevin they might leave me alone. I'll plead down to possession, do my six months, and hopefully live long enough to cash my social security checks."

"That's great. You tell me what happened so I can inform the police. That lets you off the hook, but what about me? How long is it going to take these thugs to figure out who squealed on them?"

Jack considered my question briefly. Apparently he hadn't thought that far ahead. "That's what you get paid for, isn't it?" he grumbled. "To take on the bad guys."

I was flattered. My own version of my job description had been more modest: documenting insurance fraud, catching unfaithful spouses in the act. Occasionally I had stepped into harm's way, but never intentionally.

At least until now.

"You're going to have to give me more help if you want me to go to the police. "Knowing that I represent Tommy, they're going to be more than a little suspicious if I come to them with some vague story about drug dealers killing a thirteen-year-old boy in a residential treatment center."

"I don't have anything else to give you," Jack said defensively.

"What about the person who gave you the information about Kevin's murder?"

Jack began to fidget. "I couldn't do that. They would know where the information came from."

I shrugged.

"Besides," he continued, "I don't want to get this guy in trouble. He didn't have nothing to do with it."

Such loyalty. At least he had narrowed the field. The person who gave him the information was a man. Maybe Jack would reveal more if I kept prodding him.

Before I could find out, Dr. Clover cleared her throat and spoke. "I may be able to help you."

"How?" I asked.

"I would rather speak to you privately," she said.

Jack looked at her suspiciously but did not say anything. I was reluctant to let him leave though I really didn't think he would tell me much more.

I nodded. Jack stood and zipped up his jacket. "I meant what I said before about wanting to help Tommy. He's a weird kid but he doesn't deserve to be locked up for this." He pulled on his hat, pushed back the chair and started to leave. He paused at the door and called over his shoulder, "You be careful, Doc. Don't let them mess with you."

I was moved by his expression of concern for Dr. Clover. For a second I considered telling him the truth about the state police visit to the campus. Before I could decide, Jack was gone.

"They weren't coming for us, were they?" Clover said, reading my mind.

"No. Possum Ridge has other problems."

"I was afraid of that. I feel bad for my brother, but I feel even worse for the kids and the staff. Possum Ridge used to be a first-rate treatment center. A parent could send a child here and feel assured that the youngster would get state-of-the-art treatment and consistent, nurturing care. Not as good as being at home, but for most of the kids it was the best option available. The families couldn't handle their behavior and the local agencies weren't geared up to provide the intensive therapy and support needed to maintain them in the community."

"What changed?"

"It's a complicated story. To tell it right would take more time and energy than I have. Let's just say that my brother developed some personal problems which not only diminished his capacity to lead but also impaired his judgment, especially his choice of people to help him. The day that Harrington woman was promoted, the fate of this school was sealed."

I was curious to hear her perceptions of what had happened but saw that as another story, one that had little bearing on Tommy and Kevin.

"You said you might be able to help." I noticed that she had begun to pick at her nails.

"Before, when I said I was meeting with you because Jack had been my patient . . . that was only part of it. There's another reason I was concerned when I heard the state police had come to campus. A more personal reason."

"Such as?"

"Such as the fact that fifteen years ago I was hopelessly addicted to amphetamines. I could barely concentrate enough to learn my patients' names, much less minister to their psychiatric needs. I was in debt up to my eyeballs paying for my addiction and I was on the verge of losing my husband, the one person on this earth who loves me for whom I am, not what I do for him."

Her confession took me by surprise. It was the last thing I expected to hear from this seemingly self-assured psychiatrist.

"Don't look so shocked," she said. "Even physicians can be stupid and self-destructive." Suddenly she started laughing. "Even when the empirical data looks you square in the eye and tells you that you're going to die if you don't quit."

"I don't understand what's so funny."

"Nothing really, except me. I've been beating you over the head with the club of empirical proof since the first moment you walked into my office. Now I'm telling you how, in spite of all the scientific evidence about the harmful effects of amphetamine misuse, I let myself slip to the brink of destroying my life. I know it's not funny. I guess I'm embarrassed that you know my secret."

"I . . . I don't think any less of you," I said, groping for the right words.

Clover laughed even harder. "That's a double-edged compliment if I ever heard one. A little like jumping off a ladder. If you begin at the bottom rung there's not much risk of getting hurt. I wonder what your opinion of me was before my little confession."

It was time to refocus.

"What does your addiction have to do with Kevin's death?"

"Nice move, Mr. Fenton. I can see why the Hammonds hired you." She was no longer laughing, but her smile had a devilish twinge. "Fortunately my story has a mostly happy ending, for me at least. When I was at the verge of total self-destruction, one of the nurses—we actually had two full-time nurses in those days—came to my office one afternoon. She sat down across from me, in the chair you're sitting in I believe, and offered me a choice. I could either take a leave from my position and enroll in an impaired physicians treatment program or she would go to the district attorney's office with a list of children I had treated improperly and file charges of medical negligence. She spoke kindly to me but there was no doubt about her intent. In fact, she told me that if the D.A. wasn't interested, she was certain the local newspaper would be."

"I guess she made your choice easier."

"Damn right. I was stupid, but not a total idiot. The first few months were extremely difficult. Not just for me. My husband and brother also had a tough time. I felt especially bad for Harold. He was in a difficult position."

"Jesus, he sure was." I tried to imagine how it would feel, being responsible for the treatment and safety of a group of very disturbed children while wanting to support your sister who is an excellent psychiatrist and a hard-core addict.

"Actually the toughest part for him was after I completed the intensive treatment program."

"You were recovered?"

"Recovering, recovering. An addict is never fully recovered. It's a lifelong process."

"Sorry."

"That's okay. It's a common misconception. I still go to NA meetings several times a week. And I try to work my steps every day. Because of that plus my husband's love and the courage of my brother, I'm still able to practice medicine. I consider myself blessed to be able to come here every day and work with these special children."

Dr. Clover's lower lip began to tremble. She took a deep breath, slowly exhaled, and leaned back in her chair. "Sorry," she said smiling at me. "It still gets to me."

"No problem."

"Part of what bothers me is seeing the change that has occurred in my brother during the past few years . . . and knowing there's nothing

I can do. When I completed my treatment, I came to him and asked if I could come back to work. I realized this put him in a difficult position, but I was desperate. The rehab had helped but I was still pretty shaky. Without work I didn't think I could stay clean and I couldn't imagine anyone else hiring an addicted child psychiatrist."

"What did your brother say?"

"He didn't hesitate. He said the school hadn't been the same without me and he wasn't telling me that because I was his sister. The only hitch was he had to get the Board's approval. They have ultimate responsibility for what happens at Possum Ridge, and the potential liability associated with bringing back a confirmed speed freak to practice medicine was too great. Especially since the drug addict was the director's sister. Harold felt he had to bring this to the Board."

"What was their response? The fact that you're here now makes me assume they went along with your brother's recommendation."

"Not exactly. In fact they were adamantly opposed. 'The safety and well-being of the children, the good name of the program.' The usual platitudes decision makers hide behind when they're unwilling to deal directly with their discomfort."

"What changed their minds?"

"The only thing that could have gotten them to reverse their decision. Harold submitted his resignation. At that time he *was* the program. If he left, most of the referring agencies would have stopped sending kids to the school. I suspect that some of the staff, the better ones, might have followed him."

"Pretty gutsy move."

"Yes it was. In several respects, Possum Ridge is Harold's whole life. Even more so than for me. He never married. The kids and staff are his family. I don't know what would have happened to him if he didn't have his work at the school." She paused and turned toward the window. In the pale light of her desk lamp she looked vulnerable and sad. I imagined that she was thinking of her brother and what he had become.

She began to pick at her fingernails again. "Having convinced the Board to keep me, he had to deal with a new set of risks. It didn't take a pharmaceutical genius to know that I was still fairly unstable. What if I fell off the wagon? What would happen if I mismanaged one of the children's medication? I could have brought down the whole school and my brother with it. Yes, he was pretty gutsy. And when I wake up in the middle of the night in a cold sweat, I think he was pretty foolish for taking such a big risk."

"Sounds like it all worked out."

She looked at me as if she was trying to figure out how to respond. "Not quite. It turned out there was another hitch. This one didn't work out as well."

She was dragging out her story and I began to feel irritated. "What happened?" I asked casually, trying not to reveal my impatience.

It was no use. She was too perceptive. "I'm sorry this is taking so long. It's hard for me to talk about it."

My irritation subsided immediately. It was quickly replaced by one of my most common reactions: guilt.

"That's okay. Take your time."

Mercifully Dr. Clover took me off the hook. "There was a young man. I met him at my NA meetings. He took a special interest in me. He explained to me how the meetings were conducted, told me about the significance of anniversaries, how important it was to find a sponsor to provide support and help you work the Twelve Steps. He was very friendly and solicitous, always asking me how I was, if there was anything he could do for me."

"Sounds like a nice guy."

"I thought he was, at the time. One evening, about six weeks after I started attending NA meetings, my door bell rang. I opened the door and was surprised to see him, the fellow from the meetings. He asked if he could come in, he had something important to discuss with me. I'm usually pretty careful. As a child psychiatrist it comes with the territory. But Barrett—that's his name—seemed trustworthy, so I let him in. That was my first mistake. He told me he knew where I worked and that I was on probation."

"Whoa, I thought the 'A' in NA stood for anonymous. Don't they have rules about confidentiality and privacy?"

"They certainly do, but Barrett chose not to follow them. Unfortunately it's difficult to enforce these rules. It's not like a doctor-patient or lawyer-client relationship where you can go to a professional board when you feel your rights have been violated."

"What did he want to talk to you about?"

"He reviewed, in elaborate detail, my history of drug use and my employment status at Possum Ridge. He knew things about my reinstatement that only the Board, my brother, and I had knowledge of. I still don't know where he got his information.

"When he finished the history lesson, he came to the point. He didn't want to cause any problems for me and the school. He did have certain needs however, which I could help him meet. If I helped him, the information he possessed would never find its way into the wrong hands. To make sure there was no misunderstanding about what he meant he waved a copy of the local newspaper in my face."

"What kind of help did he want?" I asked, though I was fairly confident I already knew.

Dr. Clover opened her desk drawer and pulled out a prescription pad. "He told me he had some friends who needed special medications that they were unable to obtain. If I would occasionally write a scrip for him, he would be grateful."

Watching her gouge her cuticles made me wince. I averted my eyes and waited for her to continue.

"I pleaded with him, appealed to his sense of decency. But it was no use. He's cold-hearted. He was then and he is now. He's also an active user who supports his habit by running drugs for his supplier."

"But how could he attend NA meetings? Don't you have to be clean?"

"The meetings are conducted on an honor system. The members are pretty sharp, but there's no drug screening and participants aren't required to speak. Barrett's sleazy but he's not stupid. After he 'recruited' me, he stopped coming to the meetings. I might not hear from him for three or four months. Then he would call or stop by my house. Sometimes he wanted stimulants, other times he asked for sedatives. Once he had me write a prescription for Zovirax, which is used to treat viral conditions."

"That's strange."

"I thought so. Maybe he had the flu and didn't' want to pay for a visit to his doctor. Anyway, last week he called me and said he was going to come to my house. I told him I had a late meeting but he insisted.

He seemed more desperate than usual. I agreed to see him at eleven. When he got to my house, he was quite anxious. He asked me for a glass of bourbon. When I told him I didn't have any liquor in the house he became angry. Finally he stopped yelling at me and asked me to write a prescription for Ativan. At the time I didn't understand why he wanted that medication. It wasn't until tonight, when Jack talked about Kevin's murder, that I figured it out."

"What's Ativan?"

"It's a mild sedative. The generic name is lorazepam. A fraction of a milligram can put someone out for a couple of hours. It's fast-acting and has virtually no side effects other than some post-sleep grogginess."

"Which would be hard to detect in Tommy's case?"

"Exactly."

"You really think Barrett's involved in Kevin's murder?"

"It makes sense. Barrett works for drug dealers, according to Jack. Kevin was killed by drug dealers. Jack said Tommy didn't stab Kevin, yet he was found in the same room with the knife in his hand."

"What if Jack's lying?"

"I thought of that possibility. Jack's not exactly a model citizen but he's always been honest with me. Besides, I don't think he's smart enough to concoct a story like that in order to divert attention from himself."

"What if someone else put him up to it? What if someone else wanted to divert our attention?"

Clover shrugged. "I suppose that's possible. But we won't really know until we answer a more basic question: Who would want to kill Kevin and why?"

"I can't answer that question. But there is an interesting coincidence that I'd like to pursue. Jack said the drug group that moved into this area is from central New York. Tommy is from Onondaga County which is in central New York. So was Kevin."

Clover stood and walked to a file cabinet next to the door. She pulled out a drawer and after a brief search removed two thick folders. She opened each folder to a green sheet of paper. She scanned both pages, closed the folders and returned them to the file cabinet.

"As you know," she said, "Tommy's from Liverpool. Kevin lives in Eastwood, which, if I'm not mistaken, is several miles from Liverpool."

"That's right. Eastwood is part of the city of Syracuse. Liverpool is a suburb to the north. Is there anything in the folders that suggests the boys knew each other before they came here?"

"No. Tommy was in a special education class. Kevin hardly ever went to school. It's unlikely that their families had any contact. Before DSS took custody, Kevin lived with his mother, who was on welfare. As far as I can tell the father wasn't in the picture. The foster homes Kevin was placed in were all in the inner city. It's unlikely the boys or their families came into contact with each other."

I stood up and stretched. "Sounds like a dead end. I don't think we're going to find a connection between Tommy and Kevin. At least not in Onondaga County." I began to pace. "That leaves the boys and the drug dealers. I doubt there's a link between Tommy and the central New York narcotics group. Now we just have to figure out if Kevin . . . "

"Marty," Clover interjected, "why are you smiling?"

I didn't realize I was smiling, but it didn't surprise me when she pointed it out. This was the part of investigative work I really liked. Figuring out the puzzles, especially the difficult parts. Most people became frustrated when they reached an impasse, when they have no clues or leads, nothing tangible to pursue. Not me. I thrive on frustration, the intellectual kind that is. I'm weird that way.

"I'm sorry, Just a personal quirk. I get excited when I begin to narrow down the possibilities."

Now it was her turn to smile. "Would you like to talk about these feelings of excitement?" she said with a wry grin. "Besides, at this moment the possibilities seem so narrow that they're virtually invisible to the naked eye. But maybe I'm being too much of an empiricist."

It was nice to know the doc had a sense of humor.

"I guess you're right," I said. "We don't have any leads, not even a narrow one. But I'm encouraged by Jack's story. At least we know Tommy didn't kill Kevin. Now we just have to find a way to convince the Northampton legal establishment that he's innocent."

"I like your positive attitude, Mr. Fenton."

"I like it better when you call me Marty."

"Okay, Marty. And you can call me Abigail. Since we're being so familiar with each other, why don't you move your butt out of here and try to find out what the connection was between Kevin and the drug dealers. I'll call Jack tomorrow, see if I can coax some more information from him."

"Fair enough. Faith Pasternak, Tommy's lawyer, has been doing some research on the boys and the staff. I'll call my friend in the Syracuse Police Department. Maybe he can shed some light on the group from central New York pushing drugs in this area."

I waited while Dr. Clover packed her briefcase. She closed up the office and walked downstairs to the parking lot. To my surprise Dr. Clover stopped at a red Saab convertible and unlocked the door. I had expected something more conservative, a Ford Taurus or a Buick Skylark. She turned the key in the ignition and the engine started. She pulled out of the parking space, drove a few feet, and stopped. She rolled down her window and stuck her head out. "Be careful, Marty. These are not nice people."

I watched her drive off and wondered why someone as smart and competent as she was would become involved with drugs. My graduate courses in social psychology didn't offer any help in answering that question. Maybe I would have to break down and take a course in clinical psych.

The sky was still mostly clear, but occasionally a cloud would pass through, covering the moon and casting an eerie shadow on the school's buildings. I thought of all the children who had resided at Possum Ridge. What was it like for them, living away from home in this beautiful but restrictive setting? Did they appreciate the care they were given? Did they feel that the therapeutic interventions they received actually helped them cope with their problems? Or were they unable to get past the pain of their disability, the resentment they felt for being ejected from their homes and communities?

I could feel the presence of these lost souls; not just the children who currently lived at Possum Ridge, but those who had been there earlier. I could feel their presence but I didn't know what they were thinking or feeling.

A large cloud passed in front of the moon. I don't believe in ghosts but at that moment I felt like a child on his first visit to a haunted Halloween house. It was exciting to be there but I wanted to get out as quickly as possible.

As I drove away from Possum Ridge, I wondered where Ollie was at that moment and realized I hadn't thought of her for a couple of hours. Was I so engrossed in my work or had I finally put my relationship with her to rest?

I didn't have a chance to address that question. As I came around a curve, I saw a beam of light and a cloud of smoke in the wooded area on my right. I pulled to the side of the road and peered through the windshield. The light was coming from the headlamps of an automobile.

I jumped out of my car and hurried down the slight incline. The automobile was a Ford pickup truck. And the cloud of smoke was steam rising from the radiator which had proven to be less resilient than the oak tree around which the front of the truck was wrapped.

Peering through the driver's window I saw a single passenger, a man slumped over the steering wheel. I pulled him out of the car and laid him on the ground. I put my fingers to his neck but there was no pulse. I was about to start CPR when I noticed blood trickling down the back of his head. When I turned him over, I realized that CPR wouldn't help him.

Jack Liddy had a large hole in the back of his head.

CHAPTER TWENTY-ONE

I'm sorry mommy. I'm sorry. I won't do it again.
Bring me home. Please bring me home. I'll be good. I promise.
I hate it here. The kids make fun of me. The staff aren't nice.
They make me do things I can't do. You don't make me do
those things. Please bring me home. I won't do it again. I'm
sorry.

It was one of the few times I wished I carried a cell phone. I tried to flag down a passing car but at that time of night there was no traffic. Then it struck me that whoever had done this to Jack might still be in the area. If his demise had anything to do with Kevin's murder, they might be interested in adding me to their list of victims.

I ran to my car and pulled open the door. Before I got in, I looked in the back seat, fearing that someone had sneaked in while I was attending to Jack. Finding no one I jumped into the car and immediately locked all the doors.

I considered driving back to Possum Ridge to use a phone, but the idea made me nervous. What if Jack's killer had gone to the school looking for Dr. Clover—or me? I drove toward Northampton. About two miles up the road I found a convenience store that was open. After repeatedly assuring the clerk that I wasn't going to make a long-distance call, he let me use the phone behind the counter.

The police came quickly. Two no-nonsense officers checked Jack and confirmed that he was dead. While the younger policeman called the medical examiner, the other officer asked me to repeat my story. He didn't like that I was a private investigator and was even less pleased that I knew Jack and wasn't willing to give them any information on how he fit into the case I was working on. I decided to postpone that conversation until Faith and I could meet with Darrow, the assistant district attorney.

After giving me the usual warnings to not leave town and be sure to call them if I remembered anything that might be relevant, they finally let me go. I was worried that I might miss Ollie but decided it would be wise to drive within the speed limit.

As I drove past the convenience store I noticed a pair of bright headlights in my rearview mirror. I wondered if I was being followed, but stopped worrying when I slowed down and the car passed me.

It was after ten when I reached Northampton. Even at that time the streets were filled with people. Most of them looked like students engaged in intense conversation or fooling around the way students do when they've had too much to drink. I had trouble finding a parking place but got lucky when someone pulled out of a spot just as I drove into the metered lot behind the stores and restaurants on Main Street.

Walking toward the street, I noticed how quiet it was. I began to walk more quickly. I heard footsteps behind me but when I turned I couldn't see anyone. I started running. In the distance a woman laughed and I instinctively slowed my pace. I could hear myself breathing and felt foolish.

Suddenly someone pushed me hard against a car. "Make a sound and I'll slit your fuckin' throat," my assailant hissed, as he pressed the flat side of a knife blade against my throat. A second man grabbed my arm and bent it up behind my back. I held my breath and waited, hoping I wouldn't cough or hiccup or do something else that would give them reason to perform surgery on my neck.

"How's it going, Mr. Fenton?" The voice belonged to a third person. There was something familiar about it, but I couldn't identify who it belonged to. "Got yourself in quite a mess, haven't you? You shouldn't meddle in other people's business. It can be hazardous to your health."

A vague image formed in my head: a noisy crowded place, people milling around, the room rotating. I began to feel dizzy. The image shifted and came into focus. Now I was standing in front of a urinal being bombarded with loud bowel sounds.

The man holding my arm pivoted me away from the car. Fortunately his knife-wielding partner synchronized his turn well. I wondered if they practiced this move.

Standing in front of me was Barry, the clean-cut, congenial detention-home worker and part-time student. He still looked clean cut but the scowl on his face and arms folded across his chest did not communicate congeniality. "I thought you were a smart fellow, Fenton. With all of your graduate training and detective experience I was convinced you'd be able to figure out your services weren't wanted here."

"What the hell's going on?" I asked angrily. "Did you shoot Jack? Are you the one who killed Kevin?" The goon increased the pressure of the blade against my neck. I decided to forego further inquiries.

"Good questions," Barry said. "You should have saved them for your thesis. That would have been more productive—and safer."

I weighed my options. I could continue to confront Barry and risk having my throat slit. Or I could take a more subtle approach and wait them out. I could listen to what they were saying, try to figure out what they were up to. And hope they wouldn't slit my throat while I prayed for divine intervention.

Not much choice there.

I opted for compromise. I would engage them in conversation but in an oblique non-confrontational manner, lulling them into a false sense of security. When they dropped their guard I would gently coax the truth from them.

"Any good restaurants in this town?" I asked, appealing to their gastronomical sensibility.

"Shut the fuck up, asshole," the arm twister replied, spraying saliva into my ear. "Talking about food makes me hungry and when I'm hungry and there's no food I get real mean."

So much for oblique.

Barry stepped forward and poked his finger at my chest. "You've put us in a bad position, Fenton. We had this situation under control. The police had their suspect. We didn't have to hurt anybody else. It was back to business as usual and everything was cool."

"Except for Tommy Hammond," I blurted out, instantly regretting that I had spoken. The hungry one yanked my arm up hard and Barry punched me in the stomach. I doubled over, pain shooting through my arm and shoulder. Mercifully the goon let go of my arm and pushed me

215

to the ground. I lay there, trying to catch my breath, cradling my arm, wishing I was someplace else.

"We can't leave him there," Barry said. "Somebody's going to come along and get suspicious."

"What do you want us to do with him?" This time it was the man with the knife. "We could drop him in the Connecticut River. Nobody would find him for months."

"No," Barry responded. "We need to find out what Jack said and whether he or Fenton spoke to anyone besides Doc Clover."

"I'm going to enjoy this," the arm twister said, rubbing his hands together in anticipation.

The threat of being tortured terrified me. These guys were not playing. At the same time my concern for Dr. Clover, whom they would surely go after next, and my anger at them for setting up Tommy to take the blame for Kevin's death were escalating. These feelings were so strong, in fact, that they actually pushed aside the fear I was experiencing and filled me with a sense of outrage. The terror was still there, I'm sure, but it was being smothered by these other feelings.

The pain in my shoulder was beginning to subside and my breathing had returned to normal. I considered what to do next.

I knew I was no match for them physically. Any one of my captors could easily overpower me. I had seen a knife and I was fairly certain they had at least one gun. If I was going to get out of this alive I would have to rely on my brain power. How I was going to do that was not clear to me.

There was one other possible scenario but that didn't seem likely. Ollie, sensing that something was wrong, would come looking for me. Finding me sprawled on the ground in the parking lot, surrounded by three thugs, she would spring into action, vanquish my assailants and carry me off to safety. She had done this before, so why not now. It sounded good, but even in my current state of delusion I knew an Ollie rescue was highly improbable. For all I knew, she wasn't even thinking about me at the moment.

"Let's get him out of here," Barry said. The other two men, both of whom were considerably larger than me, reached down and pulled me up by my arms. Holding me between them as if they were supporting a friend who had too much to drink, they carried me along the row of parked cars until they came to a large black van.

"This is the van you used to run us off the road after you left the detention center, isn't it?" I said to Barry.

He smiled.

"You probably did the same thing to Jack before you shot him." The arm twister started to bend my arm but Barry motioned him to stop.

"You're taking this too personally, Fenton," Barry said. "These are simply business transactions. Sometimes it's necessary to take appropriate action to protect one's financial interests. Shopkeepers install security systems, large corporations reduce prices to undercut their competitors; even nations are sometimes forced to intervene to defend their economic interests."

"So you're admitting you killed Jack." I was desperately trying to buy time. I was thinking as hard as I could but wasn't having much luck.

"I won't make a statement without my lawyer present," Barry said. He was smiling again and I wanted to smash his face.

As the sadistic pair began to lift me into the van an idea formed in my tired brain. Granted it wasn't a great idea, maybe not even a good one. But it was all I had. "You don't think I left Clover's office without calling someone to pass on what Jack told me, do you?" I was counting on them not knowing whether Jack revealed their names to me before he died. I assumed Jack pleaded for his life before they shot him, swearing he hadn't told me who he was working for. They, of course, had no reason to believe he was being truthful.

"Just who might you have told?" Barry said, toying with me.

I was ready for his question. "I told Faith Pasternak, Tommy's lawyer. By now she's passed on the information to the police and the district attorney's office." Calling Faith was a good idea. Too bad I hadn't thought of it at the time.

"And I suppose the cops will be swooping down on us any second," Barry said. He was still cocky, but I thought I heard a hint of concern in his voice.

"I don't know about that. But if anything happens to me the police will certainly know who's responsible."

Barry laughed. "Nice try. If we, in fact, did kill Kevin and Jack as you suggest, snuffing you wouldn't make any difference. If we're caught and convicted we'll already be spending the rest of our lives in prison."

I had never heard anyone refer so directly to my demise. Being snuffed sounded so impersonal. I didn't like it.

Barry opened the driver's door and climbed up into the van. "You guys sit with him," he said, pointing to the back seat. My escorts hauled me into the van and closed the side door. My last vestige of hope was rapidly fading.

There was a tapping sound on the driver's window. "What the fuck," Barry said, nearly banging his head on the ceiling of the van. He turned toward the window and the color drained out of his face. "Shit," he said, rolling down the window a few inches.

"Hello, Barrett." The voice was familiar. I leaned forward and was thrilled to see the round, fleshy face of Dr. Clover. I was even happier when I noticed two blue uniforms move into view. "How's your NA program going?" Clover asked. "Working your steps?"

"Now, Doc," Barry—or Barrett—said. "You know the program's confidential. I can't really discuss that subject with all these people around us."

"Okay, fella," one of the police officers said. "Outta' the van and move real slowly."

I felt a cold metal cylinder pressed against my temple. Then I heard a click. "I'm afraid I can't do that," Barry said. "My business associate is pointing a Sig Sauer nine millimeter revolver at Mr. Fenton's head. My associate is a very competent individual but he requires a lot of supervision. Without my constant oversight there's no telling what he might do."

The officer who had not spoken craned his neck to look through the windshield. He turned back to his partner and nodded. The officer who had first spoken, a small gray-haired man in his mid- or late fifties, asked Dr. Clover to move away from the van. Then he stepped into the space she had occupied and spoke to Barry in a soft, calm voice. "We can work this out. Let's not do anything foolish. We're going to work with you." He held up his hands. Maybe he wanted to show he had nothing up this sleeve. I'm not sure. They didn't cover that in my private investigators correspondence course.

"Okay," Barry said. "Let's start working together. The first thing we need is a clear path out of here. I want you to contact the local police, the sheriff's office, the state police, and any other friggin' law enforcement group that might be interested in us. Tell them to give us a three-hour head start. No tails, no roadblocks, no helicopter surveillance. Nothing. After that they can do whatever they want. Just so they know if anyone interferes with us we will express our displeasure in a way that will not make Mr. Fenton happy."

"When will you let him go?" the gray-haired policeman asked.

"Within twenty-four hours," Barry responded. "If your guys keep their end of the deal."

"How do we know you won't blow him away?" the other policeman asked.

"It's not to our advantage. We don't need any more trouble than we already have. He's lucky there are so many eye witnesses who can place him in our van."

I didn't find the question or the answer terribly reassuring.

The two policemen conferred with each other briefly. "I'll be back in a minute," the older policeman said. "I've got to get clearance. It shouldn't be a problem." He moved out of sight. I assumed he was going to use the radio phone in his patrol car.

"Were you serious?" the arm twister whispered to Barry. He must have needed even more supervision than his partner. He didn't get to handle the knife or the gun. "Are we really going to let this joker go?"

Barry glared at him. I couldn't tell if he was reprimanding his subordinate for asking the question or expressing disdain for the man's ignorance and gullibility. How could he even consider the possibility they would set their captive free. Naturally I favored the first interpretation, but that wouldn't surprise anyone.

I heard several voices outside the van. The loudest voice was pleading with the others not to let the three men take me with them. That voice belonged to Dr. Clover and she was making a convincing argument that these were not trustworthy individuals. The other voices, the police officers I assumed, were trying to calm her down. I heard something about not wanting to rile up my captors, the decision was out of their hands, they had to play it by the book. Clover was not persuaded by their logic. She explained that she was a trained observer of human behavior

219

and could provide empirical data supporting her contention that these were dangerous men who had no intention of letting me go.

The officers were not impressed. Dr. Clover's protests became quieter and quieter until I could barely hear her. The gray-haired policeman appeared at the driver's window. Barry rolled down the window a few inches. The gun was pressed harder against my head.

"We've got the go-ahead," the officer said. "Everyone sits tight for three hours. They're aware that you're serious about your threat and they don't want to jeopardize Mr. Fenton's safety. You can leave whenever you're ready."

"One more thing, Officer," Barry said.

"Yes."

"Dr. Clover. We'd like Dr. Clover to come with us. Her psychiatric skills might come in handy. She can help keep Mr. Fenton calm, that kind of stuff."

"That's not part of our deal," the policeman protested.

"Look at it from our perspective," Barry said. "No offense to Fenton, but he's not a valuable piece of collateral. He's not a local, doesn't even live in the Commonwealth. The authorities might not care much about sacrificing him in order to take us down. On the other hand, Doc Clover is one of your own, a respected member of the medical profession and an upstanding citizen of the community."

Talk about speaking out of both sides of your mouth. One minute he's threatening to expose her as a substance abuser, the next he's nominating her for sainthood.

I could see the gray-haired policeman shaking his head. "Don't push your luck. You're lucky my superiors approved this arrangement. They're not about to put anyone else at risk. We're following the book on this one. Everybody cooperates, nobody gets hurt."

There was that book again. Why didn't the police officer volunteer to take my place? That was in the book, wasn't it? At least in every hostage movie I've ever seen. And speaking of the book, since when did the police give in so easily to the criminals' demands for a clean getaway, especially when they were holding an innocent bystander at gun point? They must be using a different book in the Pioneer Valley.

Barry didn't seem fazed by the policeman's denial of his request. He shrugged and said, "We're outta' here." He turned the key in the ignition, the officer stepped away from the van, and he backed the vehicle out of the parking space.

When the van was pointing toward the exit to the parking lot, Barry floored the accelerator and the van leapt forward. We hadn't gone a hundred feet when an automobile shot out of a parking space into our path. Barry slammed on the brakes and the three of us in the back seat lurched forward.

Within a few seconds there was a loud metallic sound behind us as the rear door was ripped from its hinges and flew away from the van. I turned to see two men in gas masks leap into the rear of the van. They each tossed a small canister into the vehicle. At first I thought they were grenades, but as soon as I saw the thick vapor escaping I knew it was tear gas. While the two guys in the back were trying to figure out what was happening, I dove over the seat onto the floor. From there I rolled over as fast as I could until I fell out of the van. Two burly officers picked me up and when they realized I was too puny to be one of the bad guys they hurried me away from the action, to the edge of the parking lot.

It was over in less than a minute. A dozen masked and armed police officers charged the van and easily subdued my three captors, who apparently hadn't planned for a tear gas contingency.

Seeing the three thugs in the hands of the police gave me considerable pleasure. I was especially happy to watch the arm twister coughing violently and crying out in pain as he tried to rub the tear gas out of his eyes. As for Barry, he didn't look nearly as sinister handcuffed to two officers, tears and mucus running down his face. I hoped it was the first of many indignities he would suffer in his new career as a prisoner.

Other than a slight burning sensation in my eyes and a scraped knee I was unscathed. Except for the uncontrollable tremor that ran through every muscle of my body. I attributed that to the trauma of my experience rather than the acrobatics of my escape and considered it a small price to pay for such a horrendous experience. With any luck I would probably stop shaking in two or three years.

CHAPTER TWENTY-TWO

Stop it. My head hurts so much. Please stop. I can't stand it.
My head is going to explode.

As Dr. Clover and the gray-haired policeman approached me, I heard someone call my name. I turned toward the group of onlookers who had gathered at the edge of the parking lot. There must have been fifty people being held back by a small cordon of police. I spotted Lars, who towered above the others. Standing next to him was Ollie, waving frantically to get my attention.

I felt both embarrassed and exhilarated. I've never liked being the center of attention. It always makes me feel as if I have to do something, to perform. When I was in the fourth grade, Mrs. Krantz cast me in the lead role in the Thanksgiving pageant. Just as Miles Standish was about to offer his prayer of thanks to the pilgrims who had gathered to celebrate surviving their first year in the New World, I panicked. The well-rehearsed lines flew out of my head and I stood quivering on the stage, filled with dread, wishing I were dead. I can't remember if I actually peed in my pants, but I do recall Mrs. Krantz, who was not a large woman, picking me up and carrying me off the stage. Since then I've tried to keep a low profile.

In spite of my discomfort at being surrounded by a crowd, I felt good. I had come through my ordeal with no more than a sore shoulder and a pair of scraped knees. Jack's killers had been caught and hopefully we would be able to prove that Barry and his thugs had also murdered Kevin. Wouldn't it be great to tell the Hammonds that Tommy had been cleared? While it would be a slight exaggeration to say I had single-handedly brought the killers to justice, it might not have happened without me.

And how about that daring escape from the van?

Oozing machismo, I puffed myself up, turned toward Ollie and raised my arm in a sign of triumph. Ollie waved back, but it seemed to me that her greeting fell short of a hero's welcome.

"Are you okay?" Dr. Clover said, putting her hand on my shoulder.

I was tempted to exaggerate my injuries but resisted. "Yeah, I'm okay. I was pretty nervous for awhile but it seems to have worked out all right."

"Yes, it did." Clover turned to the gray-haired policeman. "Sergeant Hopson and I had a small disagreement on strategy. I thought that his approach was too risky. Fortunately you were not harmed."

Hopson stuck out his hand to me and said, "You did great, Mr. Fenton. Our only concern was that you might panic and do something foolish. You came through like a trooper."

Trooper Fenton. Has a nice ring. Doesn't require a dissertation, does it? "Thanks. I have to confess that I was thrown for a loop when you let them go so easily. I thought you'd spend more time negotiating with them."

Hopson shook his head. "You've been watching too much TV. Some departments use that philosophy. Try to wear down the hostage holders. Figure they'll either get tired or realize they're not going to get away. The problem is that some of these guys, when they see they're not going to get their jet to Venezuela, they decide to go out in a blaze of glory. That's when people really get hurt."

"So you move in quickly."

"Each situation is unique," Hopson responded. "We assess what's happening: the people, the circumstance. Then we decide which strategy is most likely to work. Sometimes we wait, sometimes we move in."

"And tonight?" I asked. "What did your assessment tell you?"

Hopson looked at me for a few seconds before he responded. "Based on Doc Clover's description we decided we were dealing with a bunch of loose cannons." I wondered if he was including me in his large munitions metaphor. "The way they killed that guy in the pickup, we were afraid they might get impatient, might do something really stupid if they thought we weren't cooperating."

Suddenly I began to perspire. "To me?" I said, gulping.

6 2 23

Hopson nodded.

"What about the back door of the van? How did you do that?"

"A little state-of-the-art technology," Hopson said, giving me a conspiratorial wink. "We just got this new armored vehicle with these super magnetic pulleys. You attach the magnetic plates to whatever you want to displace, then you reel in the cables to which they're attached. They say you can rip off the door to a bank vault using this device. Our rapid response team had never used it before. They figured it was a good time to try."

I was not reassured.

"Don't look so worried, Mr. Fenton. Everything worked out okay."

I looked over at Dr. Clover and saw she was crying. Unsure of how to respond, I pulled a handkerchief from my pocket and offered it to her.

"Thanks," she said, dabbing at her eyes. "It's just hitting me. I must have been in shock." She blew her nose. "I'll clean it and get it back to you. I'm glad you're okay."

It had taken me a moment to figure out she was talking about Jack. The image of him slumped over the wheel of his truck with a bullet in his head resurfaced. It was not a pleasant picture and the fact of Jack's death was unsettling. But it was hard for me to fathom anyone becoming that upset over Jack's dying.

Again, Clover seemed to read my mind. "Jack had some undesirable attributes, but he was basically a decent person. He had some bad breaks growing up and he definitely came up short in the gene pool. Still, he had some positive qualities. I've seen him hang in there with some pretty tough kids. I guess he identified with them."

This didn't sound like the same Jack I knew, but I wasn't about to argue with her. "How did you know where to find me?"

"After you left, I started to worry about Jack. It was clear from what he said that he was mixed up with a mean crowd. Given what he knew about Kevin, I was afraid he might say or do something that would get him in trouble. His judgment wasn't very good. I tried to call him, but his phone had been disconnected. Probably didn't pay the bill. Anyway, I was driving to his apartment when I came across his truck ... and his body. The officer told me you had found Jack and had driven toward Northampton."

"But how did you know to come looking for me?"

"It didn't take a genius to figure out you might be in trouble. If they suspected that Jack was revealing their secrets, it wouldn't be difficult for them to figure out he was talking to you and me. I knew they found Jack. How hard would it be to locate you, especially since you had stumbled across Jack's body?"

I had been somewhat shortsighted. No doubt about it. "Weren't you frightened?" I asked. "You were just as big a target as me."

Dr. Clover smiled. "Considerably bigger, I would say."

"Seriously. You must have known you were in danger. You saw what they did to Jack."

She looked at me, then lowered her eyes. "Things are different now." Her voice was barely more than a whisper. "For a long time I believed that I was conducting my life according to a set of rational principles. All I had to do was gather the facts, analyze them, and apply logic. I could master any situation; not just at work, but in my personal life also. Even after I became addicted, I believed my rational mind was always in charge." She chuckled at some private joke and shook her head.

"That's a pretty high standard," I said, thinking that my batting average for rational behavior was closer to two-fifty.

"Yes. It's also an incredibly stupid, not to mention unrealistic way to try to lead your life. My recovery helped me realize how self-delusional I've been. The events of the past few days—Kevin's death, Tommy's arrest, Jack's murder—have made me even more aware of the futility of logic in matters of importance. All of my education, all of my intellect didn't help one bit. They didn't prevent these tragedies; they didn't help me understand why life is so unfair; they didn't even offer me the smallest degree of solace . . ."

"We've gotta move on, Doc," Sergeant Hopson said, pointing to a small group of people walking in our direction. "The crime scene team is going to be scouring this area and they get pretty cranky when they find civilians on their turf."

We followed Hopson as he walked toward the street. Most of the onlookers had left, but Lars and Ollie were still standing on the sidewalk. "Do we have to hang around?" I asked.

"Nah," Hopson replied. "We got a pretty good look at what went down. It's getting late and I'm sure you want to get some rest. We can fill in the details in the morning. Leave me a number where we can contact you."

In the commotion I had forgotten about Tommy, locked up in the detention home, not knowing what the hell was happening. "What about Tommy Hammond, the boy accused of killing Kevin Landry? Will he be released tonight?" As soon as I asked I knew it was a dumb question. Where would he go? What would I do with him? I had a hard time communicating with kids who were developing normally. They made me nervous and I think I did the same to them. I wouldn't have a clue about how to take care of Tommy. Doc Clover could probably arrange to bring Tommy back to Possum Ridge, but that wasn't my call to make. I wasn't sure the Hammonds or Onondaga County wanted Tommy to return there after this ordeal.

"I don't think we can do anything about that tonight," Hopson said, reminding me how dumb my question had been. "His parents and lawyer can work that out in the morning."

A terrible thought popped into my head. What if Barry had done something to Tommy? If the thugs had even the slightest worry that Tommy might be able to implicate them in Kevin's death they wouldn't hesitate to hurt him. I asked Sergeant Hopson if he would call the detention center to check on Tommy. He gave me a funny look, then sauntered off toward his patrol car to make the call.

Standing with Dr. Clover, I felt awkward. I wanted to find out why she had put herself in jeopardy in order to find me. Yet I didn't want to add to her discomfort. She seemed so vulnerable at that moment.

As always, she didn't disappoint me. Before I could resolve my dilemma she said, "I guess what I'm trying to say is I was worried about you. I had a terrible feeling that the people who killed Jack were the same ones who murdered Kevin. I had a gut feeling that Barrett was involved." She paused for a moment and grinned. "I guess I am moving away from my empirical habits."

"Yes, you are," I agreed.

"I knew they would come after you. If they found you, they wouldn't hesitate to kill you. Logic told me it was foolish to try to find you. In addition to the risk there were other practical considerations. I didn't know where you were going. I didn't even know what kind of car you drive. But I knew I had to find you. That was all that mattered at the time. I ignored all the voices of reason in my head that were urging me to be cautious, and listened to the small insistent voice which kept telling me to get into my car and go."

And for that I was grateful. "How did you know where to find me?"

"I didn't. I got lucky. I remembered you had mentioned you were going to meet some friends in Northampton. I drove downtown where all the restaurants and bars are and began to drive up and down the main streets. The kids call it cruising, I believe. When I drove by the parking lot I saw three men standing over someone. I wasn't certain it was you, but I didn't want to take a chance. Fortunately I had my cell phone, so I called the police."

For the second time that night I understood the practical benefit of modern communication technology. I wasn't prepared to run out and buy a pager and a cell phone but I would certainly think twice the next time I was inclined to curse the recorded message on my professor's voice mail.

Dr. Clover glanced at her watch. "I better be on my way. I've got an early appointment and I want to be at the school early to see what happens now that Harrington and her crew are gone."

She was looking for a graceful way to leave and the least I could do was to honor her wish. But I still had some unfinished business. I put my arms around Dr. Clover and hugged her. Her body stiffened and then she allowed herself to relax. I turned my head and whispered into her ear, "Thank you, Abigail. Thank you for saving my life." Then I kissed her on the cheek.

"I was glad I was able to find you," she said, raising her arms to my back and squeezing me. I glanced up and saw Ollie with a puzzled look on her face.

I watched Dr. Clover walk to her car and was grateful that we had moved beyond the intellectual sparring we had engaged in the first time I visited her office. Before she left, I agreed to give her phone number to Mr. and Mrs. Hammond. She wanted to meet Tommy's parents and, if they were interested, share her views on what kind of treatment might be best for Tommy once he was released from detention.

As I walked to where Ollie and Lars were standing I tried to clear my mind. I was sick of dealing with violence and corruption. I was hungry and I was tired. More than anything I wanted to have a cold beer and a thick, juicy steak, then crawl into a large comfortable bed.

I recounted the evening's events to Ollie and Lars, emphasizing my heroic feats, such as the daring escape from the van. I downplayed the terror I felt when I realized Barry and his cronies intended to kill me, but they were probably perceptive enough to figure out that it wasn't a pleasant experience.

When I finished, I suggested we get something to eat. Lars said he was tired and was going home. I considered responding to him the same way I had to Dr. Clover, but decided I wasn't yet that liberated.

Ollie and I walked along Main Street looking for an open restaurant. Most of the eating places had closed for the night. The wind picked up and it began to rain. We stepped into the doorway of a small restaurant with red checked table cloths. The menu posted on the door was simple: sandwiches, salads, a few pasta dishes. I looked at Ollie for a reaction. She shrugged. The rain was coming down harder and the prospect of finding a good steak at that time of night was not good. I opened the door and we stepped inside.

A small, balding man with hair combed across the top of his head walked toward us. Only two tables were occupied: a two-top with a young man and woman who appeared to be more interested in each other than their food, and a large table with a group of women involved in an animated discussion. I thought they might be getting ready to close, but the man greeted us cheerfully and showed us to a table in the back, away from the other diners.

After giving us a moment to look at the menu, the small man took our order. He was a congenial fellow who told us to take as much time as we needed. I couldn't tell if he had a genuine desire to satisfy his customers, even when it inconvenienced the staff of the restaurant, or if he was taking advantage of an opportunity to delay going home.

Ollie ordered a cup of hot tea and a Greek salad. I asked for a cheeseburger, fries, and a Sam Adams. If I couldn't get steak, at least I would have my beer.

The Sam Adams was cold and the cheeseburger was surprisingly good. It was my second burger and fries of the day, the first having been consumed ten hours earlier at the diner with Gloria Harrington. I don't usually load up on cholesterol, but this had been an unusual day. Ollie picked at her salad. She seemed to be preoccupied, but I was too busy wolfing down my cheeseburger to ask what was bothering her.

Against my better judgment I ordered dessert, marble cheesecake that the host, who doubled as our server, claimed was baked on the premises. I knew I would have trouble sleeping after this heavy meal, but I figured self-indulgence was in order after such a harrowing day. I offered Ollie a little and, as I expected, she declined. No problem. The cheesecake was as good as promised and I had no difficulty finishing the large wedge.

As I was pushing the empty plate away from me, Ollie said without warning, "I don't think we should see each other anymore."

My reaction, or I should say my lack of reaction, surprised me. Even a couple of days ago such a proclamation would have sent me into a tailspin: shortness of breath, head feeling like it had become detached from my body, lots of anxiety, a healthy dose of self-doubt and obsessing over why this was happening to me. But tonight was different, I didn't respond in my usual manner.

"Okay," I said, taking a swig of beer. "That makes sense."

It may have been my imagination but I thought I saw Ollie furrow her brow slightly. Surprise? Bewilderment? Disappointment? I didn't know what she was feeling but I was fairly certain this wasn't going the way she expected.

"Okay, then," she said. "I guess that's settled. Okay."

We chatted for awhile; small talk about Northampton, Ollie's reunion with Lars, my desire to get back to Syracuse to work on my thesis. I continued to be impressed by my casual response to Ollie telling me that our relationship was over. I wasn't yet ready to admit that I had reached the same conclusion but wasn't prepared to say it aloud. I wasn't being too hard on myself, however, for not being fully actualized. I had definitely made progress.

I excused myself and went to the men's room. I peeked under the stall to see if there was another unexpected occupant. Finding no one on the toilet, I walked to the sink and splashed water on my face.

The shock of the cold water released something inside me. All of the feelings I had held in check rushed to the surface. I struggled to hold them back, fearing they would overwhelm me, but they were too powerful. The day had been one long emotional roller coaster ride. My mental sparring match with Gloria Harrington at the diner. The bittersweet collapse of the Possum Ridge administration. These events, which would have provided enough excitement for a normal day, were mere speed bumps compared to the steep plunges that followed. The meeting with Dr. Clover and Jack, the first real breakthrough in proving Tommy's innocence, triggered hope and excitement, feelings that were quickly pushed aside when I found Jack's dead body on the side of the road. I barely had time to register the horror of Jack's death when I was forced to consider the real possibility that I might meet a similar fate at the hands of Barry and his henchmen.

My rescue had left me with a great sense of relief and exhilaration, admittedly heightened by my somewhat grandiose perception of my own contribution to that event. My poignant encounter with Dr. Clover, following my rescue, had also left me with a good feeling.

Even Ollie's Dear John pronouncement hadn't fazed me.

I had been able to hold everything together. Granted, I was probably in shock from the moment I saw Jack slumped over the wheel of his truck. Still I kept going and, for the most part, had done pretty well.

Now, standing at the sink, water dripping from my face, the dam burst and my feelings gushed out. My first instinct was to try to contain them, to pull them back inside. I quickly realized that wasn't going to be possible. So I let them flow. Sobs racked my body and tears carried the jumbled torment of anger, fear, and sadness to the surface.

After a few minutes the torrent of feelings subsided and I stopped crying. My emotional well was drained. That I was exhausted didn't surprise me. The toll taken by the events of the day would have worn down a stronger person than I. What surprised me was the feeling I was left with after my catharsis.

What I felt at that moment was relief. It was as if I had unloaded a huge weight, a metal ball that had become lodged in my gut. The ball was filled with my worries, my anxieties, all of the things that had weighed heavily on me for the past few months: finishing my thesis, finding out if Tommy Hammond had killed Kevin Landry, figuring out what was happening between Ollie and me. Even the events of the past few hours, discovering Jack Liddy with a bullet in his head and my sudden abduction and rescue, had expanded the size of the ball. Now the ball was gone, except for the fragments of my unfinished thesis, and I was relieved. The reality of no longer being with Ollie had caught up with me and I was feeling sad. But I knew it was the right decision and that gave me some consolation. I wiped my face with a paper towel which I crumpled it into a ball and tossed over my shoulder. Then I watched it sail in a high arc and land in the center of a waste basket a good ten feet away.

Ollie was not sitting at the table. She had left a note and a ten-dollar bill. Her note was concise and cordial:

> Sorry there wasn't a better way to do this. I don't want
> to hurt you. I'll be staying with Lars tonight. Will call you in
> the morning about return trip. Glad you cleared your client.

My response tank was empty. The note was, at that moment, nothing more than a bunch of words. I didn't even react to the part about Ollie staying with Lars. I stuffed the note in my pocket and called for the check.

I was bone weary and ready for bed. But I was not yet finished. I still had a couple of calls to make.

I considered looking for a phone booth. The prospect of spending more time in my dreary motel than I absolutely had to didn't turn me on. Standing on a dark street corner with a telephone pressed against my ear wasn't appealing, either. Especially after my encounter with Barry and his buddies.

It was a tough decision, but I hadn't lost all sense of reason. Dreary and boring prevailed over dark and dangerous. I walked to my car, which was still in the parking lot where I had been abducted, and drove back to the motel.

Faith picked up before the second ring. She sounded as if she had been sleeping.

"It's Marty. Sorry to bother you."

"That's okay. I was having a bad dream."

"Maybe this will help. Tommy's innocent. He didn't kill Kevin Landry."

"What?" She was awake now.

"Barry, or Barrett, whatever his name is. The young guy from the detention center. He's involved in drugs. He did it."

"Marty, I don't understand anything you're saying."

I took a deep breath and tried to compose my thoughts. Then I recounted, as best I could at one A.M., what had transpired since I said goodbye to Faith that afternoon in the Possum Ridge parking lot. I described my meeting with Jack and Dr. Clover, and what I had learned about the drug dealers and their involvement in Kevin's death. I told her how I found Jack with a bullet in his head; how I had called the police, then made the foolish mistake of driving into town. I gave a brief account of the events in the parking lot in Northampton, modestly understating my daring escape from the van.

The only thing I didn't share with Faith was my Dear John dinner with Ollie.

When I had completed my story, Faith asked how I was doing. I told her I was a little tired but okay. It was only a white lie. I was tired, after all.

She congratulated me for clearing Tommy. I told her I hadn't done much, which was mostly true. We went back and forth for awhile, Faith praising my accomplishments and I downplaying my role. We soon grew weary of that exchange and Faith said she would call Darrow first thing in the morning. She explained that she would have to contact the Onondaga DSS since they had custody of Tommy, even though his parents were now in Northampton. DSS would have the last word on where Tommy would go after he was released from detention. She had spoken with Mrs. Hammond earlier that evening. They had discussed what might happen to Tommy and his mother said she wanted to bring him back to Syracuse if that was possible.

I told Faith I appreciated all that she had done for Tommy. She laughed and said she was too weary to argue with me about who had done what for whom. She said she would see me in her office at nine the next morning and told me to get some sleep.

My next call also woke up its recipient, only Lou DeSantis wasn't nearly as understanding as Faith had been. After he finished berating me for calling at such an ungodly hour, I told him about the central New York drug dealers, Barry/Barrett and Kevin. He asked me Kevin's last name and when I told him it was Landry, there was a sound at the other end of the line, like someone slapping his forehead with the palm of his hand. This was followed by a series of profanities. When he had exhausted his vocabulary on select body parts and functions, which was more extensive than I imagined, Lou shared with me the source of his consternation.

He explained that a ne'er-do-well named Sean Landry had gotten behind on some gambling debts. His creditors, who didn't work in a bank but did believe in giving debtors a second chance, offered Sean the option of performing certain services in order to pay off his debt. Landry, who had an affinity for the bottle as well as the ponies, became a courier for the organization to which he owed money. His assignment was to deliver narcotics to the organization's clientele, collect payment, and return to his designated sales manager.

"You think Sean is related to Kevin?" I asked.

"Could be."

"And this fact is somehow relevant to Kevin's death?"

"It's plausible."

"Any thoughts on what might have happened?"

"How many times have I told you? Police work is a scientific endeavor. We don't rely on thoughts or hunches. We utilize state-of-the-art research methodology to gather and analyze potential evidence and develop potential hypotheses. But you psychologists wouldn't know about that."

"Okay, Einstein. Why don't you break out the microscope and start analyzing?"

"I'll make some calls," Lou said with a yawn. "Call me in the morning. I should have a better idea how the pieces fit together by then."

"Pleasant dreams," I said, grateful that Lou hadn't asked me about Ollie.

I hurried through my nighttime bathroom routine and got into bed. Ordinarily I don't have any trouble falling asleep. After what I had been through that day I expected to nod off as soon as my head hit the pillow.

My body was willing but my brain wasn't ready. The events of the day passed through my mind's eye like a slide carousel revolving on a projector. The showdown at Possum Ridge, Jack lying dead in his truck, my unpleasant ordeal with Barry and his nasty crew. As soon as I pushed one scene out of my consciousness it was replaced by another. The touching farewell scene with Dr. Clover. My late night dinner with Ollie.

With each new image I became more agitated.

I picked up my puzzle magazine and started to work on an anagram, but I couldn't concentrate. I tried counting sheep, then unicorns. I pulled the Gideon Bible from the drawer of the night stand. None of these distractions worked.

After forty minutes of futile activity I changed strategies. If I couldn't fall asleep at least I could use my time constructively. I opened my suitcase, extracted a copy of my thesis and returned to the bed. I turned to the results chapter and began to review the statistical procedures I was using to analyze my data.

In less than two minutes I was sound asleep.

CHAPTER TWENTY-THREE

The big man told me I don't have to stay here anymore. I must have been good. Maybe daddy will get me and take me home in his car.

By the next morning the rain had stopped but the pain in my shoulder had not. I aimed the shower head at the tender area but neither the temperature nor the pressure of the water was sufficient to provide relief.

I took three ibuprofen and set out for Faith's office.

Faith greeted me with a warm smile and held up her arms. I leaned down and hugged her. She drew my head into the soft spot where her shoulder and neck met. She had a faint scent of flowers on her skin and I lingered for a moment, enjoying the fragrance and warmth of her neck.

"I talked to Darrow," she said, bringing me back to the real purpose of our meeting. "He says we can take Tommy whenever DSS tells us where they want to place him. I called their emergency number and I'm waiting to hear from a supervisor."

"Have you talked to the Hammonds?"

"Yes. Mrs. Hammond called about a half hour ago asking for directions. I was going to wait until we were all together to tell them about Tommy, but my exuberance got the best of me. This is more than I can say for Mrs. Hammond. Her reaction was kind of odd."

"How so?"

"She didn't seem at all excited when I told her Tommy had been cleared. She told me that was great news and thanked me for helping Tommy. But there was no emotion in her voice. No happiness, no relief, nothing. It was like I had told her I was giving her a fifty-cent discount coupon for her favorite dish detergent."

"Maybe she was in shock. She's been so worried about Tommy. She and her husband were pretty pessimistic, especially since they felt so helpless, having given up custody. The reality of his exoneration may not have sunk in yet."

Faith shrugged and guided her wheelchair to a small conference table at the other side of her office. She picked up a thin folder. "I researched this custody transfer thing. It seemed outrageous that the state would make families give up custody of their children in order to obtain services. I didn't see how it could be legal. Turns out it isn't, at least in New York. It used to be but the legislature changed the law when they realized families were being split up for no good reason."

"You mean the Hammonds shouldn't have had to give up custody of Tommy? Did DSS mislead them?"

"Worse than that. They were given a choice: Sophie's choice, you might say. The Hammonds knew that Tommy needed intensive treatment, treatment that cost several thousand dollars a month. As long as the Hammonds retained custody of their son, he remained a low priority for DSS. The Hammonds could retain custody of Tommy and not be able to get him the care he needed. Or they could obtain the treatment he needed by giving away their only son. "

"Some choice."

"Yeah," Faith said, slamming down the manila folder. "And there isn't even a bad guy you can go after. The DSS people don't like the practice any more than you or me. They just don't have any other way to get access to funding. I suppose you could blame the politicians. They're the ones who set the budget. When you get right down to it though, the good citizens of our community would probably throw them out of office if they raised taxes to help kids like Tommy."

There was a knock on the door. Faith wheeled herself over, opened the door and greeted the Hammonds. Mr. Hammond shook Faith's hand then strode to where I was standing. He gave me a big smile and squeezed my hand forcefully. Mrs. Hammond, who looked as if she had lost her son rather than gotten him back, walked past us without as much as a nod of recognition to the small conference table on which Faith had just slammed her file folder.

It didn't take a genius to observe that something wasn't right.

Faith gestured for us to sit while she brewed some tea and coffee. Mr. Hammond took the seat to my left and Mrs. Hammond sat on my right. After she had gotten everyone their drinks, Faith summarized what had happened during the past few days, ending her account with a description of her phone conversation with the district attorney earlier that morning. When she had finished, she asked the Hammonds if they had any questions. Larry Hammond thanked us for all that we had done, telling us if it hadn't been for our efforts, Tommy would still be locked up awaiting trial for murder. He appeared to be genuinely grateful, but his exuberance seemed forced.

When Ruth Hammond said she didn't have any questions, Faith reached for a pen and pad of paper and asked, "What do you want to do with Tommy? I realize he's still technically in the custody of DSS, but you should be the ones to decide where Tommy goes after he's released from detention. If you want him to stay at Possum Ridge, Dr. Clover has promised to look after him. If you don't want him to go back there, I'm sure we can find another good residential treatment center. Of course the ideal would be if the agencies in Syracuse could put together a program for Tommy in your community, but I don't know if that's feasible now. Would you want him to come home with you?"

There was a brief period of silence. Larry looked down at his clasped hands. Ruth looked at him as if she expected him to say something. When he didn't, she turned to Faith and said, "Tommy will be coming home, but not with us." She was still looking at her husband but now I could see that it was not a friendly gaze.

"What Ruth means," Larry said, speaking to his hands, "is Tommy will be returning home with Ruth . . . but I won't."

"Why don't you tell them why you won't be coming with us?" Ruth said sharply, glaring at her husband.

Larry shook his head slowly, but didn't say anything.

"Never mind," Ruth said, dismissing him with a wave of her hand. "Why should I expect you to act differently now?" She took a deep breath and exhaled. "I can't believe I was so stupid. You live with someone for years, you think you know him. But you don't. You don't know anything . . ."

"Ruth, you don't have to do this," Larry pleaded.

"Be quiet," Ruth snapped. "You had your chance to speak. Now it's my turn." She turned away from Larry and spoke to Faith. "He goes on a lot of trips. Buffalo, Albany, New York City. Sometimes he's gone two or three days. I didn't like it, but I got used to it. When Tommy lived with us it was harder. Since he's been away, it hasn't been so bad."

I glanced at Larry. Slumped in his chair, head bowed, staring at his folded hands he reminded me of Tommy. He was a pitiful sight.

"Wednesday night I got a call from his boss, wanting to talk to him about a presentation he was supposed to make the next afternoon. I told him Larry was in Albany until Thursday morning, at least that's what he told me. His boss acted real surprised. Said he thought Larry had a noon meeting in Albany but was supposed to be back in town by late afternoon. When I repeated what Larry told me about having to stay over in Albany, his boss backed off, said he may have been mistaken.

"When he came home the next night, I confronted him. How come his boss said he was returning to Syracuse Wednesday afternoon? At first he played dumb, said his boss must have misunderstood. I wanted to believe him but I had this nagging doubt I couldn't shake. I kept at him until finally he broke down and admitted he hadn't been in Albany. He told me he'd spent the night at Arlene Sadlow's apartment and it hadn't been the first time.

"I was stunned. Arlene works at GE. Before she was divorced, she had dinner at our home with her husband. She was always friendly to me. I never suspected anything."

Larry cleared his throat. "I never meant to hurt you." I couldn't tell if he uttered these words as an act of contrition or merely wished to interrupt, if only temporarily, Ruth's painful account of his infidelity.

Ruth started to say something but changed her mind. She clapped her hand over her mouth, closed her eyes, and began to rock back and forth in her chair. Faith looked at me for guidance. The only response I could manage was a feeble shrug.

Sensing that further discussion would not be helpful, Faith told Ruth she would be talking to DSS later that morning and would contact them as soon as she worked out the details of Tommy's release to her. When Faith had finished her explanation, Ruth stood up, shook hands with

Faith and me, thanked us for our help and left. She did not look back.

Larry remained in his chair. He was no longer looking at his hands. His gaze was fixed on the chair Ruth had recently vacated. Occasionally he moved his lips, but he didn't speak.

Finally I asked, "Is there anything I can do for you, Mr. Hammond?"

He looked around as if he were not sure who had spoken. "No," he said, shaking his head. "No. There's nothing more you can do for me." With considerable effort he pushed himself out of his seat and walked over to Faith. Holding out his hand, he said, "I'm sorry you had to witness this. I wish I could give you a reasonable explanation for my behavior, but I can't. I am grateful for what you, both of you, have done for Tommy. He's been saddled with a lot of injustices. His disorder, having to leave his family to get treatment, being accused of killing this boy and not being able to tell someone he didn't do it. And now he's got to suffer again because of my stupidity. It isn't fair."

Larry continued to hold Faith's hand during his brief soliloquy. When he became aware of this, he seemed embarrassed. He gently extracted his hand and awkwardly patted her wrist. He turned to me and stuck out his hand. I shook hands but quickly removed my hand from his grasp. He offered a forced smile and thanked us again. Then he walked out of the office.

Watching Larry Hammond leave, I was painfully aware that Tommy wasn't the only one who had suffered. Ruth and Larry had both been worn to the breaking point by the seemingly endless series of crises and disappointments they had endured. Their family had been torn apart and their marriage had ultimately been destroyed. It was difficult to know how they would have fared without the added burdens they had to deal with: Who knows if their marriage would have survived? One thing was clear, however. The system they had to work with, the professionals and agencies that made them jump through so many hoops to get services for Tommy, didn't help. Their odds would have been a helluva lot better if the service system that was supposed to assist children and their families had been more rational, more compassionate.

But that was not the case. They had been chewed up and spit out by the system that promised to help them. In what seemed to be the latest and most ironic in a long series of cruel jokes that had been played upon the Hammonds, they had regained their son but lost their family.

Neither Faith nor I had much to say after the Hammonds left. As I was getting ready to say goodbye the phone rang. It was a supervisor from Onondaga County Social Services and she told Faith she had sent a fax to the district attorney authorizing him to release Tommy to the Hammonds. Faith called Darrow, who said the family could pick up their son at two o'clock.

I told Faith I wanted to be there when Tommy was released from the detention center. We agreed to meet in front of her office at one-fifteen so we could get to the detention center early, in case there were any last-minute complications.

As much as I enjoyed Faith's company, I wanted to be alone at that moment. Our meeting with the Hammonds had put a damper on our celebration. We had cleared Tommy so he could return to his family. Now he only had half of a family to return to.

My work as an investigator had shown me how unfair life can be. Being a graduate student in psychology hadn't made me any less skeptical. There was still a part of me, though, that wanted to believe that stories have a happy ending.

I walked down Main Street, trying to put myself in Tommy's place. What was going on in his head? What would he do when he saw his parents? How would he react when he found out he was going home without his father? I found I simply couldn't imagine myself in Tommy's place, and trying to think about him was giving me a headache. I needed a distraction.

I went into the first bookstore I came to and walked through the aisles, picking up books with interesting titles. I even stopped at the psychology section, but didn't find any inspiration for my thesis.

In the philosophy section I picked up a book by Nietzsche. I thumbed through the thick tome looking for something that might help me make sense of what had happened to the Hammonds, or at least distract me from the depressing thoughts I was having at that moment. Toward the back of the book I came across an interesting line: "That which kindles the lightning must for a long while be a dark storm cloud."

It didn't help me make sense of the Hammonds' awful situation and I doubted the quote would give Ruth, Larry, or Tommy any solace. It was a good quote, though. Might even be relevant to my situation with Ollie.

Eventually hunger overtook me. I went back to Pinocchio's for a couple of slices of pizza and a Snapple. I still had fifteen minutes before I was to meet Faith. I stopped at a pay phone and dialed Lou's number.

"Captured any more bad guys, Marty?" Lou said, picking up on the first ring.

"How did you know it was me?"

"Who else do I know with a western Massachusetts area code?"

"Huh?"

"Caller ID. I had it installed last week. I got tired of the solicitation callers. Especially the computer calls."

"You know how I feel about impersonal communication devices. I won't even buy an answering machine. But isn't caller ID just another electronic gimmick?"

"Ah, my good friend, I'm afraid you've fallen victim to the flawed logic of the postmodern Luddites. It's not the technology itself that compromises the integrity of our human identity. Rather it is the manner in which we actualize our core beliefs through our everyday actions that define our bond with humanity."

"Nice vocabulary, Lou. Angie must have enrolled you in another philosophy course. What did you find out about Kevin Landry?"

"I thought you'd never ask. It turns out that Sean Landry, the guy I mentioned to you yesterday, is Kevin's father. Sean was involved with one of our larger narcotics enterprises. He wasn't a major player; delivered product, collected receivables, sort of a middle man. At least he was until last November."

"What happened to him?"

"The government executed a hostile takeover of Sean's division. He and four of his colleagues were outplaced to the state's correctional facility in Attica. The pay's not as good, but you can't beat the job security."

"How long's he in for?"

"He won't be back in the marketplace for awhile. The prosecutor tried to get him to turn on his supervisors, but Sean did the math and figured it was better to spend fifteen to twenty in prison than be forced to take early retirement by one of the firm's downsizing consultants at Attica. When he refused to cooperate, the prosecutor went after him with a vengeance. He's doing eighteen years, with little chance of parole."

"So it's possible the drug dealers knew Kevin."

"Possible."

"But you said Sean didn't rat on his bosses. They wouldn't have any reason to harm his son."

"Unless they were afraid Sean was planning to make a post-sentence deal."

"Why would they kill Kevin? I could see them hurting him to send a message. But killing Sean's son sounds drastic. In fact, it might even backfire."

"I agree. But you're assuming Sean is a normal father who puts his child's well-being above everything including his own. From the little I know about this guy I'm not sure that assumption is warranted. He's an alcoholic and probably a crack addict who beat his wife before he left her with a couple of little kids and no money."

"You think he sacrificed his kid to save his own ass?"

"I don't know. I want to do some more checking. How can I get in touch with you?"

"I'm leaving Northampton this afternoon. I should be back in town this evening. I'll call you tomorrow. Say hello to Angie for me."

"I will. How's Ollie?"

I hesitated before responding. "She's fine." Which as far as I knew was true. It was I who wasn't doing so well and he hadn't asked about me.

Faith and I were the first to arrive at the detention center. It didn't look less dreary than it had on our first visit, but knowing that we would be removing Tommy from its dull confines blunted my negative reaction.

We breezed through the security clearance. The guard who had given Faith a hard time during our initial visit tried his best to be pleasant. Though it was unlikely he would ever be a serious contender for employee of the month, he did allow Faith to bypass the metal detector archway. We were escorted to a stark gray room with a rectangular table and six wooden slat-back chairs. The chairs and the table were bolted to the floor, which made it impossible for Faith to sit at the table. She parked her chair in the center of the wall facing the long side of the table and I stood next to her.

In quick succession, Ruth, Darrow, and Larry were escorted into the room. Because their divorce was still pending the court required approval from both parents in order for Ruth to take custody of their son. Then Tommy was brought in by a thin pale man in a brown suit who introduced himself as Mr. Jackman, the superintendent of the detention center. He asked everyone to sit at the table. The Hammonds, Darrow, and Jackman sat. Faith declined politely and I remained at her side.

Tommy seemed even more gaunt and disheveled than when I had first seen him. His hair hung down over his eyes and his clothing was so baggy it looked as if it might fall off of him.

Tommy didn't give his parents any sign of recognition when he first entered the room. Once seated, he looked at his mother, who sat at one end of the table, then at his father at the opposite end. From where I was standing I could see his face clearly. His expression revealed neither anger nor pleasure. He seemed to be looking for an explanation, wanting his parents to tell him what was happening, where he would be going. Unable to seek answers with his voice, he relied on his eyes to gather information.

For the next twenty minutes, he shifted his gaze back and forth between his mother and father, not uttering a word until the final moment of the meeting.

Darrow began by apologizing to the Hammonds for Tommy's arrest and incarceration. He tried to cast the incident as an unfortunate though unavoidable mistake. Larry nodded politely during the D.A.'s recitation; Ruth seemed more interested in Tommy, smiling at him, trying to lock onto his constantly moving eyes. When Darrow was convinced he had done everything in his power to deter the Hammonds from suing the county, he shifted gears. He reported that he had received a letter from the Onondaga County DSS authorizing Tommy's release to his parents. The letter, which had been faxed to him that morning, stated that the Hammonds' decision to withdraw Tommy from residential treatment and bring him home nullified his eligibility to receive funding from the Department of Social Services. Therefore, they were transferring custody back to his parents. The DSS supervisor added that the department stood ready to assist the Hammonds if, in the future, they were in need of services, and offered the family her best wishes. Darrow told the Hammonds they needed to sign a release terminating the voluntary custody arrangement with DSS.

Mr. Jackman tried to reassure the Hammonds that Tommy had been treated well in his facility, but nobody seemed interested.

Sensing that Ruth was becoming impatient, Faith asked if there were any other matters that needed to be discussed. Darrow said they were free to take Tommy whenever they were ready. Then he asked casually what they planned to do with Tommy.

Ruth, who had been gathering her belongings, stopped abruptly and turned toward Darrow. "What are we going to do?" she said, glaring at the D.A. "You've got a helluva nerve asking me that. You certainly had a clear idea about what you wanted to do with my son. Lock him up and throw away the key. Or did you want to go all the way and ask for the death penalty?"

"Ruth," Larry said, trying to intervene.

"Stay out of this. You've already done enough." She turned back to Darrow and said to him, "Now that Tommy's no longer a candidate for your trophy case, he's no longer your concern. The fact is you don't give a damn what happens to him."

"Mrs. Hammond," Darrow said. "You've got good reason to be upset."

"Damn right I do," Ruth snapped. "More than you know."

"I know our department contributed to your anguish," Darrow said. "But we were just doing our job."

Ruth glared at Darrow. "Okay. You want to know what we're going to do with Tommy. I'll tell you. I'm going to take him back home with me and pray to God he doesn't tear our house apart or worse. Yes, I know he can be violent. But it's not because he wants to. He can't help it. And without the proper treatment he's not going to get better. So Tommy and I will go back to our house and try not to get on each other's nerves while we wait for someone to figure out how to help him. I don't know when that will be or what it will be, but I'm certain about one thing: I will not give Tommy away, again. Not to social services, not to some residential treatment center, not to anyone. He's staying with me."

I looked around the room. Only Faith and Tommy were looking at Ruth. Faith looked as if she were on the verge of crying. Tommy stared impassively at his mother. I wondered what his troubled mind was thinking.

Ruth picked up her bag and coat, and squeezed out of her chair. "Let's go, Tommy. We're going home."

Tommy remained in his seat until Jackman took him by the arm and guided him out of the chair. Ruth walked to her son and put her arm around his shoulder. At the door Tommy stopped and turned back to the table. He hesitated for a second, then said in his high-pitched voice, "My daddy."

Larry waved awkwardly and started to get up. Before he could get to his feet, Ruth nudged Tommy toward the door. He did not resist.

We waited until Jackman escorted Ruth and Tommy to the lobby. When Jackman returned, Larry asked if he could use the telephone to call a taxi to take him to the bus station. I thought of offering him a ride to Syracuse with Ollie and me, but decided that wouldn't be a good idea. Jackman took Larry to an office with a phone. In the lobby Darrow asked why Larry wasn't going with his wife and son. Faith told him she didn't want to talk about it. She promised to call him later. He shrugged, thanked me for helping to solve the case, and left.

As I walked with Faith to her van, I thought about what we had been through during the past few days. Seeing Tommy, so frightened and vulnerable in that awful detention center. Being run off the road on the way back to Northampton and learning about the terrible accident that claimed the lives of Faith's husband and young son. At first I had felt sorry for her. But watching her work, negotiating with the assistant attorney general for information on the investigation at Possum Ridge, setting up the confrontation between Prosic and Harrington and the Board members, my attitude quickly changed. It was not just her intelligence and shrewdness that impressed me. Even more striking than her ability to figure out how to get what she needed was her courage.

I hadn't yet figured out whether it was in spite of or because of her disability, but she was without a doubt, one tough lady. From the moment she told the guard in the detention center she would scratch out his eyes if he laid a hand on her, I knew she was a person to be reckoned with.

And then there was her compassion. She really cared about Tommy. Not just as a client, but as a frail, helpless child who needed someone to stand up for him; someone to look out for his interests as the cold, efficient justice system that had locked him up and all but thrown away

245

the key rushed to record another closed case on its tally sheet.

Tommy had needed someone to care for him, to believe in him even when there wasn't a shred of evidence to support his innocence. Faith had been there for him from the moment she laid eyes on him and had stayed with him throughout the entire awful ordeal.

Sure, I was there, too. But my involvement wasn't as personal, wasn't as intense, especially in the beginning. Tommy's parents were my clients and my job was to get information on what had really happened at Possum Ridge. It was Faith's passionate advocacy that raised my level of involvement; raised it to the point where I cared about what was happening to Tommy. Without her, Tommy might still be sitting in that drab concrete block room in the detention center.

Faith pushed the button to release the van's hydraulic lift. As the platform slid to the ground a wave of anxiety overcame me. My heart began to beat rapidly and I was having difficulty breathing.

Faith looked at me and asked, "Is something wrong?"

I took a deep breath and shook my head. "I'm just tired," I said, unable to tell her that I didn't want to say goodbye.

She smiled and turned her chair toward me. "You didn't think you were going to get away without giving me a hug?" she said, lifting her arms toward me.

I bent down and embraced her. The scent of flowers was still there and I could have stayed there all day.

After a moment she patted me on the back and said, "You've got a lot of energy for a tired guy. Do you mind easing up a little before I suffocate?"

I quickly let go of her and stood up, nearly falling over in the process. "Sorry," I muttered.

Faith was still smiling. "I've really enjoyed working with you, Marty." 'Me, too."

"Maybe we'll try it again. You never can tell." She rolled her chair onto the platform, secured her brake and activated the lift.

As I watched her ride up and disappear into the van, her words echoed in my head: You never can tell, you never can tell. I was filled with an odd sense of sadness and hope.

CHAPTER TWENTY-FOUR

I'm happy I'm home. All my games and things. Just where they're supposed to be. My room smells nice. Mommy made me pancakes. Where's daddy?

The trip back to Syracuse couldn't have been worse. I considered taking the bus but that seemed cowardly and immature. Besides, I was running low on cash and after paying the motel bill the credit line on my VISA card was maxed out.

It wasn't that Ollie was mean or hostile. She was actually quite civil. She wanted to know about my meeting with the Hammonds and asked several times during the trip if I wanted to stop for something to eat or to use the restroom.

The problem was not what was being said. The problem was figuring out what to talk about and the discomfort we both felt trying to avoid any reference to our broken relationship.

We spent the four-hour drive in virtual silence, Ollie's eyes fixed on the road ahead of us while I pretended to enjoy the surrounding scenery. Occasionally one of us would initiate a superficial conversation about the traffic or the weather, but these awkward attempts to ease the tension ended as abruptly as they began.

The only positive thing I could say about the trip was that it didn't snow as we passed through Utica, though the dark cloud was still hanging over that section of the highway.

It was dark when Ollie dropped me at my apartment. She promised to call in order to make arrangements to pick up the clothing and other items she kept at my place. I began to tell her there was no hurry but caught myself, afraid my remark might be misconstrued as a signal of

247

hope about the future of our relationship.

My apartment has never been a cozy, cheerful abode. It serves a useful purpose, giving me a place to eat, sleep, and store my belongings. As long as it meets those basic needs I don't pay attention to the aesthetic qualities of my living space. It doesn't bother me that the orange and brown plaid recliner doesn't match the blue sofa or the imitation oriental rug. I don't mind that the venetian blinds are always askew or that the light fixture in my bedroom is attached precariously to the ceiling by a single loose screw. I barely notice the grime on the windows that filters out the few hours of sunlight that blesses Syracuse each month.

That night, however, the drab, discordant ambiance of my apartment depressed me. I don't know if it was the contrast to the beauty of the Pioneer Valley—though certainly not my motel room—or a displacement of my grief about losing Ollie, but I didn't like being there.

I emptied my suitcase and checked in with the answering service. To my relief, none of the regulars were on duty. The woman who answered gave me my messages without any strange mannerisms or editorial comments. My mother had left a less-than-subtle reminder that she would be turning sixty-five next month. Professor Singleton wanted to schedule a meeting to review progress on my thesis. Lou DeSantis asked me to call him.

I ignored the first two messages and called Lou. When he suggested we get something to eat, I jumped at the chance to get out of my apartment.

The Dinosaur Bar-B-Que Express is a unique eating establishment. Located on Willow Street, on the west side of the city, it draws an odd mixture of bikers, suburbanites, and university types. It is always crowded and noisy and for good reason. The barbeque ribs and chicken are out of this world.

I spotted Lou standing by the bar. He had a penchant for fine wines, a habit he had acquired from his wife Angie, but at the Dinosaur he had to settle for a Budweiser. True to his policeman's instinct, he limited our conversation to Syracuse sports until we were seated at a table. I understood the logic of his decision, but thought it was an empty gesture since the noise level was so high I could barely hear my own voice.

Just as we were about to exhaust our knowledge of local sports happenings, the hostess called Lou's name and guided us to a corner table. After we placed our orders, Lou told me what he had learned. "You remember Jerry Bullard, the guy who runs information systems for the sheriff's department?"

I nodded. "The guy who helped us with the Majorski case."

"Yeah. He owed me a favor. I asked him to find a willing accomplice to Sean Landry, someone who wouldn't mind sharing some personal information with me for a small price. He came up with Arnie Valentyne, sometime drug runner, sometime informant."

"And what did Mr. Valentyne say?"

"Interesting, very interesting. Our hypothesis about the drug bosses killing Kevin to send a message to his dad seems unsupported. Sean may not be much of a father, but at least he's not guilty of sacrificing his son to save his own ass."

"So, what hypothesis did Mr. Valentyne offer?"

"It turns out that Kevin brought about his own demise. Valentyne told me that one of the middle managers of the local narcotics organization used to have a supervisory relationship with Sean. Apparently this man even transacted some business with Sean in Kevin's presence."

"I thought Sean had deserted his family."

"He did. According to Valentyne, when Sean was flush and sober, which didn't occur often, he would take Kevin to a ball game or the circus. It was before one of these outings that Sean met with his supervisor.

"When the organization expanded into western Massachusetts, Sean's supervisor was given a promotion and sent to head up the new operation. One day Kevin ran into the supervisor. Arnie wasn't sure whether it was during a transaction at the school or while the kids were on an outing. Apparently Kevin recognized the guy and started mouthing off to him. Kevin taunted the guy, told him he knew he was a drug dealer and he was going to turn him in to the police. Arnie said the dealer was justifiably upset. The organization was beginning to do well in western Mass and he didn't want some kid to mess up their business. Arnie said the guy has a wicked temper and a good memory. He didn't like the kid threatening him and he took steps to make sure Kevin wouldn't create any more problems for him."

"He killed Kevin because he said he was going to turn him in?"

"Apparently."

"But Kevin was just a kid. Didn't he know that kids are always bragging about what they're going to do? Most of the time they don't do anything."

Lou shrugged.

"The supervisor," I asked, "did Arnie say anything about him, what he looked like, how old he was?"

"Not much. He said he was a young guy; looked clean cut, but was a real mean son of a bitch."

I swallowed hard as I considered what might have happened to me if Dr. Clover hadn't decided to come looking for me.

The server brought our dinners and we focused our attention on the large portions of messy but delicious food. When we were finished, Lou pushed his plate away and asked how Ollie was doing. Realizing Lou would eventually figure out something was wrong, I decided to tell him the truth. Lou listened patiently, making sympathetic noises as I recounted the events leading to our breakup. I was about to thank him for being so supportive when he leaned forward and said, "I'm sorry, Marty . . . I know this is hard for you. But, frankly, your bad news has helped me achieve a renewed sense of congruence."

"What do you mean?"

"I always thought Ollie was an intelligent woman. Her taste in men didn't seem consistent with the profile of a cerebrally competent person. Now that she's dumped you, my confidence in her intellectual prowess has been restored."

I reached across the table and tried to swat him but he pushed back his chair and I missed him and knocked over a glass of water. While I was apologizing to the server, Lou picked up the check. "The least I can do to support you in this time of despair."

When we were on the street, Lou put his arm around my shoulder. "I hope you understand that my biting sarcasm is really a coping mechanism I've adopted to deal with my fear of intimacy. I really feel bad for you, buddy. I'm also proud of you for getting that kid off. Hercule Poirot couldn't have done a better job."

Lou had a point. Not about Hercule Poirot, but his sardonic wit.

Sometimes I wasn't sure how to take him. Was he hiding his feelings behind his Funk and Wagnall vocabulary or was he just putting me down? At that moment I didn't have the energy to explore that question. So I thanked him for his concern and promised to go with him next week to a Sky Chiefs' game.

Walking to my car I saw a black van slow down as it approached me. The passenger in the front seat rolled down the window and my heart began to pound. I could barely squeeze out a reply when the young woman asked me directions to the Carousel Mall.

After many lively but inconclusive arguments with the grad students in clinical psychology I had finally come around to their position. I was now an ardent believer in post-traumatic stress disorder.

On the drive home I began to think about my reaction to Ollie's announcement that she wanted to stop seeing me. At the time I was surprised, even stunned, by the relief I experienced. Now, removed from the immediacy of the event, it began to make sense to me.

My desire to settle down with Ollie had less to do with who she was than my own inability to see what I was doing. Once I realized I was tired of bouncing from one relationship to another what did I do? I decided to get married. And whom should I marry? The woman I was with at the time, of course. How convenient.

No wonder Ollie was uncomfortable. She was merely a pawn in my blind rush toward marital bliss. To make things worse I didn't even have the guts to deal with my own self-deception. I left it to her to break up with me.

How could I be such a jerk, especially to Ollie who had always been straight with me?

As I backed into a parking space in front of my apartment, I considered the irony of my new found insight into my relationship with Ollie. How many times had I argued with Lou about the existence of the unconscious? He had read several books about psychoanalysis in his effort to build his vocabulary and had become a firm believer in Freud. I always took the negative position. Now that I had successfully plumbed my psyche I was filled with ambivalence. I never liked to lose a debate, but I also felt a sense of pride in my accomplishment. I was having difficulty enjoying this achievement, however. As soon as I realized why I felt relieved when

251

Ollie broke up with me, a dense emotional haze fell on me.

Self-insight was definitely overrated.

By the morning my haze had lifted and I was ready to deal with my unfinished business. I wasn't sure whether I had worked through the embarrassment and shame of the previous evening or had stored these feelings in a dark corner of my unconscious. Frankly, I didn't care as long as I didn't have to deal with them at that moment.

My first order of business was to visit Jerome Hannigan, Esquire. I wanted to let him know the outcome of my investigation and thank him for making the connections that allowed me access to Tommy and his records. I also had an ulterior reason for dropping by his office. Hannigan had gone to law school with Faith Pasternak and I was hoping to learn more about this unique woman.

The Southwest decor still seemed incongruous with the surrounding light industrial motif. Hannigan was dressed in a charcoal gray pinstriped suit that probably cost as much as the tuition for a course at the university. His crisp white shirt accentuated his tan. His red and gray necktie was a far cry from a bolo, but he still wore a silver belt buckle.

"Returned from the battlefield?" he asked, gesturing me to sit on the mauve sofa I had occupied during my last visit. "How did it go?"

I recounted the events of the past few days, beginning with my initial meetings with the county attorney and Faith, and finishing with Tommy's release from the detention center and the painful irony of the Hammond family being split up once again. I left out what had happened between Ollie and me as well as the unexpected and disconcerting feelings I had developed for Faith. Besides those two matters, neither of which I considered to be central to Tommy's case, my account was accurate and complete. Unlike my first visit to Hannigan's office, I was relaxed and fairly confident. The fact that I had not used a bogus story to get an appointment with him this time certainly contributed to my sense of comfort. Our success in clearing Tommy didn't hurt either.

When I had finished my story, Hannigan uncrossed his long legs and leaned forward. "When I first met you," he said softly, "I didn't think much of you. In fact, I almost threw you out of here. If the Hammonds hadn't been in such an awful predicament, I probably would have." He paused and I began to feel nervous. Then he grinned. "I'm glad I didn't."

"Me too," I said with relief.

Hannigan raised his eyebrows in admonishment. I had been given my turn; now it was his. "I spoke to Faith last night. She said that if it hadn't been for you, Tommy would still be awaiting trial. She thinks you're quite competent, though unorthodox. She actually thanked me for referring you to her."

I wanted to ask him about Faith but I remembered his raised eyebrows. I decided to wait for a better opening.

"It's funny," Hannigan said, looking at the wall where his diplomas and certificates hung. "When we were in school I was convinced Faith would be the next Ralph Nader or the first female Attorney General of the United States. She could have been either. She had a passionate sense of justice, an amazing grasp of the law and boundless energy. Most of our classmates were jealous as hell of her. When the recruiters from the big firms came to campus, she was always first on their list. She could have had any job she wanted."

"What about Zach, her husband? Wasn't he at the top of your class?"

Hannigan looked puzzled. "I don't know where you got that idea. Faith was number one in our class for all three years. Zach was a nice guy and he was no dummy. But he wasn't in the same league as Faith."

I racked my brain trying to remember where I had gotten the impression that Zach was at the top of his class. Hadn't Faith mentioned that her husband was number one? No, she had told me Hannigan was second, but she never actually identified who was first. Had Faith's glowing description of Zach led me to conclude that he was first in their class . . . or was I less liberated than I wanted to believe? I had assumed that the top dog had to be a man and not even considered the possibility that Faith might have had the best academic record.

Shame on me.

While I was mentally flagellating myself, Hannigan's secretary called on the intercom to tell him he had a telephone call. I offered to leave but he told me he would take it in the reception area. I would have said goodbye but I still had a couple of questions.

While I waited for Hannigan to return, I walked around the office looking at his Southwestern artifacts. In addition to the R.C. Gorman painting he had several lithographs depicting Indian life and a sand painting of a Navajo god. Indian baskets and pottery, including a beautiful black-and-white Acoma vase, were scattered throughout the office and a large metal statue of the flute-playing Kokopelli, the spirit of luck and prosperity, filled one corner of the room. As I admired Hannigan's collection, I realized how much I had learned about art from Ollie. It was one of many good things Ollie had given me, I thought sadly.

I noticed a wood-framed photograph of three people on Hannigan's desk. On one side was Hannigan, dressed in a handsome argyle cardigan sweater. A tall, attractive blonde woman stood on the other side. In the middle was a slim girl with a head full of dark braids. She appeared to be eight or nine years old and although photographs are often deceptive, she certainly had the facial features and coloring of a Native American.

"Beautiful women aren't they?" Hannigan said as he entered the room. "Fortunately Emily didn't have to rely on my gene pool for her physical attributes, though with any luck she might have picked up some of Lydia's ample good looks. All of that is beside the point, however, since our daughter, Emily, was adopted by us when she was eight weeks old."

It was interesting to watch Hannigan speak about his family. His face was softer, his voice more mellow, almost playful. He actually smiled, especially when he spoke about Emily, and his gray eyes seemed to sparkle.

"It's odd that you should be looking at that picture now," he said.

"How's that?"

"Coincidence. I'm amazed by the number of coincidences that occur." He pointed to the picture. "The same woman who made it possible for us to adopt Emily also played a big role in reuniting Tommy with his family—his mother, at least."

"Faith?"

"No." Hannigan shook his head. "Ernestine Stamwell, the supervisor at DSS who gave you my name. If she hadn't done that you never would have hooked up with Faith. I know Faith thinks the world of you, but knowing her as I do, I'm confident you couldn't have cleared Tommy without her."

My ego was bruised but he was right. And one of my lingering questions had finally been answered. Now I knew why Hannigan was so willing to help me when he found out that Mrs. Stamwell had referred me.

"That's not the only coincidence," Hannigan continued. "Guess who just called me. Your friendly local narcotics syndicate. They want me to represent the guy accused of killing Kevin Landry."

It took me a few seconds to process what he had just told me. The drug dealers wanted Hannigan, who was indirectly responsible for Barry being caught, to defend their employee when he was tried for murder. It wasn't exactly a conflict of interest, but it was strange.

"Are you going to do it?"

Hannigan did not respond immediately. The pained look on his face could have been caused by physical discomfort but I guessed that the source of his distress was more likely moral. After a moment he said, "I think so. Yes, I think I will represent him. After I graduated from law school, I lived in Boston for a few years. I took the Massachusetts bar so I can still practice in the Commonwealth."

"But after all the suffering he's caused Tommy and his family, not to mention what he did to Kevin, doesn't it sicken you?"

"It does. But the practice of law shouldn't be, can't be personal. Probably the most important thing I learned at Harvard was that our judicial system—the right to a fair and speedy trial, along with a few other fundamental rights like freedom of speech and the right to vote— is the linchpin of our democracy. As an attorney, it's my duty to ensure that every individual, no matter how reprehensible his character or deed, receives due process. Personally I might prefer to see a lowlife like this drug dealer hanged by his testicles from a telephone pole. But as an officer of the court I feel some responsibility".

I wanted to argue with him, to rebut his idealistic position on due process, to express my outrage at the possibility that a dirtball like Barry might dodge punishment for his heinous crime because a smart lawyer like Hannigan was able to outfox the prosecutor or find a procedural error in the police investigation. I wanted to yell at Hannigan for betraying Tommy and Kevin and their families and yes, even me and Faith.

I searched for the right words. When I couldn't find them, I thought of Faith and what she might have said if she were here. But it was no use. If Faith were here, she would have shared my outrage and indignation at the prospect of Kevin's killer receiving less than the maximum sentence. Then she probably would have supported Hannigan's decision to represent Barry and, if the attorneys' ethical code permitted, she might have volunteered to assist him.

Suppressing my self-righteous inclination, I thanked Hannigan for hooking me up with Faith. I repeated his assertion that I couldn't have solved the case without her. He told me he was glad I had proved his first impression of me to be wrong and said he might call on me if he needed someone to help him gather evidence on behalf of a client.

My curiosity about Faith had not been satisfied but I decided not to push my luck. Better to leave on a high note than jeopardize Hannigan's high opinion of me by asking questions that might be viewed as irrelevant. I pushed myself up from the comfortable couch and shook his hand.

I walked through the reception area and Hannigan's secretary said, "Good afternoon, Mr. Fenton. I hope you have a pleasant day."

Her use of the prefix "Mister" did not go unnoticed.

Stepping outside I was hit by a stiff, cold wind and noticed the telltale thick gray cloud mass moving in from the northwest. The question was not whether it would snow, but when and how much?

Still feeling the glow of Hannigan's praise I decided to tackle my thesis. Before going to Hannigan's office I had thrown my briefcase into the trunk of my car, hoping for inspiration. I retrieved the well-worn canvas bag and laid it on the passenger seat next to me. I turned the ignition key, breathed a sigh of relief when the engine started, and turned my trusty Honda in the direction of the computer lab.

As I approached the campus large wet flakes of snow began to drop from the sky. My uncertainty about whether this was a good or bad omen was soon erased when I found a parking place directly across from the building that housed the computer laboratory.

It felt as if I had been away for a long time, though in fact it had only been three days. The last time I had been in the computer lab Ollie paid me a surprise visit and invited me to join her for a piece of cake and a cup of coffee. This time there would be no Ollie. The couple making out in the corner of the room didn't help the growing sense of melancholy I was experiencing.

I turned on the computer and inserted my data disk. I tapped my way through a series of menus until I found the program that would give me access to my data. The results of my research appeared on the screen.

What could be easier? Select the appropriate statistical test, load in the numbers and punch the command button. It sounded so simple.

Thirty minutes later I had a knot in my stomach and was still staring at the same bank of numbers.

Maybe I wasn't sufficiently inspired.

I switched over to my E-mail. There were two new messages. The first, from my advisor, Professor Singleton, was brief:

from:msingleton@lilac.syru.edu
to:mfenton@lilac.syru.edu
subject: thesis
Marty,
          I've missed you. Call at your earliest convenience.
Sincerely,
MS

To the uninformed reader it appeared to be a polite, nondescript note. I knew better. Being familiar with Professor Singleton's penchant for understatement, I interpreted his message as an unequivocal command to get my butt into his office immediately. I was definitely in deep trouble.

I pushed the *Next* button and the second message appeared:

to:mfenton@lilac.syru.edu
from:fpasternak@gmail.com
subject: Thinking of You
Dear Marty,
          Not much has happened since you left. The three men who abducted you have been indicted. Barry has been charged with-first degree murder as well as felony distribution of class A and B narcotics. The other two were charged as accomplices. The district attorney will probably offer the two underlings a reduced sentence if they turn on their boss. I wouldn't want to be Barry's attorney.

Possum Ridge is in turmoil. Prosic, Harrington, and the other three top administrators have been removed from their positions. The Board called an emergency meeting and appointed an interim executive team. Dr. Clover—the psychiatrist—was appointed as acting director. I think she can turn the school around with the Board's help. I don't know the specific charges against Prosic and the others but I'm pretty sure they won't be members of the civilian workforce for a long time.

Otherwise things have been pretty dull. I've caught up on my paper work; even did a little housecleaning.

Hope your trip to Syracuse was okay. I miss your stimulating company.

Incidentally, I've been doing some thinking. With all of the changes taking place these days, I'm no longer convinced that age differences between people who like each other are necessarily a problem. What do you think?

Fondly,

Faith

I read the last paragraph of her message several times. When the words began to blur I switched back to the program menu and clicked on the *Open* icon. I scrolled to the file labeled thes.dat. and hit the *Return* button. Then I sat back in my chair and listened to the monotonous buzz as the computer searched for my precious data.

Suddenly I felt inspired.

Author's Note

The characters and events in this book are fictional. Unfortunately the problems, pain and frustration experienced by the Hammond's in attempting to obtain appropriate treatment for their son are not. While many of the people who work with children with mental health needs are dedicated and caring, the systems in which they function are broken.

Every day families encounter barriers as they seek help from a child serving system that is inadequate, inappropriate, irrational and often unfriendly. I have met some of these families and have learned a lot from them. Through their experiences I have become even more aware of the large gaps in service that exist, the paucity of resources allocated to child mental health and the lack of coordination among agencies responsible for serving children. I have seen how these problems affect children with behavioral and emotional challenges and disrupt the lives of their families. The dilemmas families deal with are compounded by the disappointingly high level of stigma and misconception that still exists regarding mental health, and the absence of compassion and empathy expressed by some, though certainly not all service providers. Equally striking has been the persistence and courage displayed by many of these families as they confront the obstacles in their path and refuse to give up on their children, even when their seems to be little reason for hope.

I have been fortunate to have worked with a number of people who share my interest in and concern for children with emotional and behavioral challenges and their families. Dean Parmelee, Shirley Wiley, Isaac Abraham, Jeri Baker, Donald Oswald, Bela Sood, Julie Linker, Stephanie Vitanza, Jeri Hosick, Nancy Doyle, Pat Doyle, and Melissa Hopkins have helped me to understand the dilemmas posed by the child mental health system and what can be done to eliminate the cruel practice of parents being forced to relinquish custody of their children in order to obtain help.

In preparing this book I have had excellent assistance from my editor, Larry Mazzeno and publisher, Robert Pruett.

As always, my wife, Nancy, and my adult children, Nick, Tim and Jessye have provided continuous encouragement and support as I worked on this book and have offered constructive feedback when my execution has fallen short of my intent.

For More Information about Child Mental Health:

American Academy of Child & Adolescent Psychiatry
www.aacap.org
(202) 966-7300

American Psychiatric Nurses Association
www.appna.org
(866) 242-2443

American Psychological Association
www.apa.or/topics/topicchildren.html
(800) 374-2721

Autism Society of America
www.autism-society.org
(800) 328 -8476

Federation of Families for Children's Mental Health
www.ffcmh.org
(240) 403-1901

Judge David A Bazelon Center for Mental Health Law
www.bazelon.org
(202) 467-5730

Mental Health: A Report of the Surgeon General
www.surgeongeneral.gov/library/mentalhealth/home.html

Mental Health America (formerly the National Mental Health Association)
www.nmha.org
(800) 969-6642

National Alliance on Mental Illness (NAMI)
www.nami.org
(703) 524-7600
(800) 950-6264 (information helpline)

National Association of Social Workers
www.naswdc.org/children.asp
(202) 408-8600

Printed in the United States
201345BV00003B/184-282/P